Cardiology

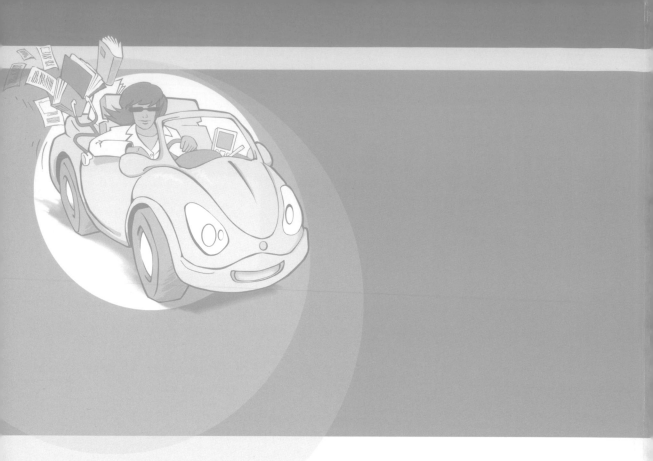

First and second edition authors:

Anjana Siva

Mark Noble

Mohamed K Al-Obaidi

CRASH COURSE

Third Edition

Cardiology

Series editor

Daniel Horton-Szar,
BSc (Hons), MBBS (Hons), MRCGP
Northgate Medical Practice,
Canterbury, Kent, UK

Faculty advisor

Adam Timmis,
MA, MD, FRCP, FESC
Professor of Clinical
Cardiology,
London Chest Hospital,
London, UK

Ajay Jain BSc, MRCP
Specialist Registrar in Cardiology, London Chest
Hospital, London, UK

Matthew Ginks BSc, MRCP
Specialist Registrar in Cardiology, St Thomas'
Hospital, London, UK

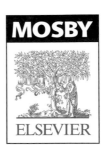

MOSBY

ELSEVIER

Edinburgh • London • New York • Oxford • Philadelphia • St Louis • Sydney • Toronto 2008

MOSBY
ELSEVIER

Commissioning Editor:	Alison Taylor
Development Editor:	Kim Benson
Project Manager:	Morven Dean
Page design:	Sarah Russell
Icon illustrations:	Geo Parkin
Cover design:	Stewart Larking
Illustration management:	Merlyn Harvey

First edition 1999
Second edition 2004
Third edition 2008

ISBN: 978-0-7234-3464-1

British Library Cataloguing In Publication Data
A catalogue record for this book is available from the British Library

Library of Congress Cataloging In Publication Data
A catalog record for this book is available from the Library of Congress

Note
Knowledge and best practice in this field are constantly changing. As new research and
experience broaden our knowledge, changes in practice, treatment and drug therapy may
become necessary or appropriate. Readers are advised to check the most current information
provided (i) on procedures featured or (ii) by the manufacturer of each product to be
administered, to verify the recommended dose or formula, the method and duration of
administration, and contraindications. It is the responsibility of the practitioner, relying on their
own experience and knowledge of the patient, to make diagnoses, to determine dosages and
the best treatment for each individual patient, and to take all appropriate safety precautions. To
the fullest extent of the law, neither the Publisher nor the Authors assumes any liability for any
injury and/or damage to persons or property arising out or related to any use of the material
contained in this book.

The Publisher

Cardiology is a fantastic specialty because it combines history taking and clinical examination with investigations which can readily be correlated with the disease process. There is great satisfaction in the often rapid improvement in the patient's symptoms following appropriate treatment. Furthermore this field is growing rapidly with new and exciting technologies. I hope that this book not only equips you with the information you need to pass your exams, but enables you to further your interest and enjoyment of cardiology.

Ajay Jain
Matthew Ginks

Is there a more exciting speciality in clinical medicine than cardiology? Advances in the prevention, diagnosis and management of heart disease in recent years have been widely reported. Lives saved by lifestyle modification and treatment of hypertension and lipid disorders together with revascularisation and secondary prevention strategies are reflected in our national statistics which show marked reductions in cardiovascular mortality over the last 20 years. Nevertheless, cardiovascular disease remains the major cause of premature death and the major challenge to clinical medicine in the 21st century, not only in western societies but increasingly in developing countries as well.

This Crash Course in Cardiology is designed to arm the reader with the knowledge base needed for a clinical introduction to this fascinating specialty. In the first part of the book emphasis is given to bedside assessment through history and examination with additional information about the diagnostic contributions made by electrocardiography, biomarkers and imaging techniques. In the second section, attention shifts to the major cardiovascular disorders, from angina pectoris to congenital heart disease, focusing on pathophysiology, clinical features, investigation and treatment. Finally, in the third section, we return to basics with a description of history taking, clinical examination and how the clinical findings should be recorded in the medical record.

Like the other books in this series, the material is contemporary, the content accessible and the coverage comprehensive. Students will enjoy reading this book and we hope that many will come to share our own enthusiasm for clinical cardiology which remains the most popular speciality among junior doctors contemplating a career in hospital medicine.

Adam Timmis
Faculty Advisor

More than a decade has now passed since work began on the first editions of the Crash Course series, and over four years since the publication of the second editions. Medicine never stands still, and the work of keeping this series relevant for today's students is an ongoing process. These third editions build upon the success of the preceding books and incorporate a great deal of new and revised material, keeping the series up to date with the latest medical research and developments in pharmacology and current best practice.

As always, we listen to feedback from the thousands of students who use Crash Course and have made further improvements to the layout and structure of the books. Each chapter now starts with a set of learning objectives, and the self-assessment sections have been enhanced and brought up to date with modern exam formats. We have also worked to integrate material on communication skills and gems of clinical wisdom from practising doctors. This will not only add to the interest of the text but will reinforce the principles being described.

Despite fully revising the books, we hold fast to the principles on which we first developed the series: Crash Course will always bring you all the information you need to revise in compact, manageable volumes that integrate pathology and therapeutics with best clinical practice. The books still maintain the balance between clarity and conciseness, and providing sufficient depth for those aiming at distinction. The authors are junior doctors who have recent experience of the exams you are now facing, and the accuracy of the material is checked by senior clinicians and faculty members from across the UK.

I wish you all the best for your future careers!

Dr Dan Horton-Szar
Series Editor

Contents

Abscess   a collection of pus within a cavity.

Accessory pathway   an abnormal connection between atrium and ventricle that is capable of propagating a cardiac impulse.

Afterload   the pressure that the left ventricle must produce to eject blood out of the heart.

Anticoagulation   treatment intended to prevent blood clotting.

Angina pectoris   commonly known as **angina**, is chest pain due to ischaemia (a lack of blood and hence oxygen supply) of the heart muscle, generally due to obstruction of one or more coronary artery.

Angiogram   is a medical imaging technique in which an X-ray picture is taken to visualize the inner opening of blood filled structures, including arteries, veins and the heart chambers.

Angioplasty   see Percutaneous Coronary Intervention.

Apex beat   the most downward and lateral position on the chest wall where the cardiac impulse can be felt.

Arrhythmia   cardiac rhythm disturbance.

Asystole   absence of contraction. Asystole is when the heart has stopped beating and is different from ventricular fibrillation where the heart is still contracting, but not in a co-ordinated manner.

Atheroma   is an accumulation and swelling in artery walls that is made up of cells, or cell debris, that contain lipids (cholesterol and fatty acids), calcium and a variable amount of fibrous connective tissue.

Atrial fibrillation (AF)   irregular contraction of the atria resulting from disorganized electrical activity, typically results in an irregularly irregular pulse.

Atrioventricular (AV) node   region of specialized conducting tissue between the atria and ventricles that functions to regulate the electrical conduction.

Atrium   one of the two (upper) collecting chambers of the heart.

Bradycardia   a heart rate <60 bpm.

Bundle branch block   This is failure of conduction in either the left (LBBB) or right (RBBB) bundle branches.

Cardiac catheterization   is a minimally invasive procedure to access the coronary circulation and blood filled chambers of the heart using a catheter. It can be used both for diagnosis and treatment.

Cardiac failure   also called heart failure, this is a reduction in cardiac pump function such that there is inadequate perfusion to metabolizing tissues.

Cardiac output   the amount of blood pumped out by the heart every minute, calculated as stroke volume (SV) × heart rate (HR).

Cardiac tamponade   compression of the heart as a result of accumulation of fluid in the pericardial space. This results in reduced cardiac output and can be fatal if untreated.

Cardiomyopathy   heart muscle disease.

Cardioversion   reverting the heart to a normal rhythm, this can be done electrically (with a DC shock), or using drugs (pharmacological or chemical cardioversion).

Central venous pressure (CVP)   the pressure of blood in the great veins as they enter the right atrium.

Contractility   the strength with which the myocardium contracts.

Cyanosis   bluish discoloration of the skin due to the presence of deoxygenated haemoglobin in the blood vessels.

Defibrillation   is the definitive treatment for the life-threatening cardiac arrhythmias ventricular fibrillation and pulseless ventricular tachycardia. Defibrillation consists of delivering a therapeutic dose of electrical energy to the affected heart with a device called a **defibrillator**

Defibrillator can be external, transvenous, or implanted, depending on the type of device used.

Dehiscence reopening at the site of a surgical closure or apposition.

Diastole part of the cardiac cycle where the ventricles are relaxed and filling.

Echocardiogram is an ultrasound of the heart. Also known as a cardiac ultrasound, it uses standard ultrasound techniques to image two-dimensional slices of the heart.

Ectopic an event occurring at a place other than its normal location, for example ventricular ectopic beats originate from the ventricles, not the sinoatrial node.

Electrocardiogram (ECG) graphic representation of the electrical activity of the heart over time.

Electrophysiological (EP) study an invasive test used for accurate diagnosis of arrhythmia and assessment of the function of the heart's electrical pathways.

End-diastolic pressure (EDP) the amount of pressure in the ventricle at the end of diastole.

End-diastolic volume (EDV) the amount of blood in the ventricle at the end of diastole; the greatest amount found in the ventricle throughout the whole cardiac cycle.

Ejection fraction the proportion of EDV which is ejected by contraction.

Heart block also called AV block, this is abnormal slowing or failure of conduction from the atria to the ventricles.

Holter monitor ambulatory ECG, usually attached to the patient for 24–48 hours.

Hypertension high blood pressure.

Hypertrophy increase in the size of a tissue or organ resulting from an increase in cell size.

Hypotension low blood pressure.

Hypoxia low oxygen levels.

Infective endocarditis infection of the endothelial surface of the heart by a microorganism.

Ischaemia lack of blood supply to a tissue.

Infarction tissue death caused by inadequate perfusion.

Laplace relationship a relationship between the tension, pressure and diameter of a container (implied blood vessel), as Tension = Diameter × Pressure.

Left ventricular failure is a condition that can result from any structural or functional cardiac disorder that impairs the ability of the heart to fill with or pump a sufficient amount of blood through the body.

Mean arterial pressure the average pressure in the system at any point in time, approximated as the diastolic pressure + (1/3 × pulse pressure).

Myocardial infarction a medical condition that occurs when the blood supply to a part of the heart is interrupted, most commonly due to rupture of a vulnerable plaque.

Ohm's Law a relationship between resistance, pressure and flow inside a container (implied blood vessel), as Pressure = Flow × Resistance.

Pacemaker an area that leads to cardiac electrical activation; this may be natural (intrinsic, such as the SA node) or artificial, e.g. a permanent pacemaker.

Percutaneous coronary intervention (PCI) commonly known as **coronary angioplasty** or simply **angioplasty**, is a therapeutic procedure to treat the stenotic (narrowed) coronary arteries of the heart found in coronary heart disease.

Perfusion movement of blood through an organ or tissue.

Pericarditis is an inflammation of the pericardium (the fibrous sac surrounding the heart).

Precordium the surface of the lower anterior chest wall.

Preload the pressure and volume experienced by the heart before contraction.

Radio frequency ablation (RFA) the use of radiofrequency energy to create a therapeutic burn, intended to treat cardiac arrhythmia.

Shunt flow of blood through an abnormal communication between chambers or blood vessels. This may allow blood to flow between the pulmonary and systemic circulations.

Shock a situation where insufficient blood flow is reaching the body's tissues, causes commonly described as hypovolaemic, cardiogenic or septic.

Sinoatrial (SA) node the impulse-generating (pacemaker) tissue located in the right atrium.

Sinus rhythm a rhythm under direct control from the sinoatrial node.

Sphygmomanometer a device used for measuring blood pressure.

Starlings Law a phenomenon whereby the heart increases its output by increasing its strength of contraction when the fibres of the myocardium are stretched.

Stent is a tube that is inserted into a natural conduit of the body to prevent or counteract a disease-induced localized flow constriction. Often used in PCI (see above).

Stroke volume (SV) the amount of blood ejected from the left ventricle with each beat.

Stroke work (SW) the amount of external energy expended in one ventricular contraction. SW is the arterial pressure (AP) multiplied by the SV.

Supraventricular literally "above the ventricle" i.e. originating from the atria or AV node

Syncope temporary loss of consciousness from reduced blood flow to the brain.

Systemic vascular resistance (SVR) the resistance to blood flow offered by all of the systemic vasculature, excluding the pulmonary vasculature. It is calculated as (MAP – Right Atrial Pressure) / CO.

Systole part of the cardiac cycle where the ventricles are contracting.

Tachycardia a heart rate >100 bpm.

Torsades de pointes literally meaning "twisting of the points", this is a form of ventricular tachycardia in which the complexes are polymorphic (i.e. have variable shape).

Total peripheral resistance (TPR) the resistance to the flow of blood in the whole system. It is calculated as arterial pressure / cardiac output.

Troponin is a complex of three proteins that is integral to muscle contraction in skeletal and cardiac muscle, but not smooth muscle, damage to myocardial cells leads to an elevation in the plasma troponin level.

Vasodilatation increase in the calibre of a blood vessel.

Ventricular relating to the heart's ventricles (pumping chambers).

Ventricular fibrillation (VF) irregular uncoordinated contraction of the ventricles, fatal if untreated.

THE PATIENT PRESENTS WITH

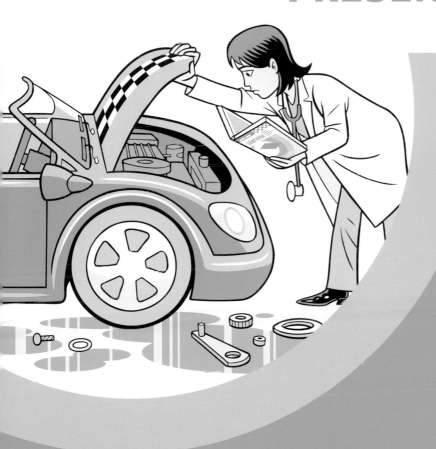

Objectives

By the end of this chapter you should:

- be able to take a clear history from a patient presenting with chest pain
- be aware of the differential diagnosis of chest pain
- be able to examine the patient with chest pain
- understand the appropriate investigations for a patient presenting with chest pain.

DIFFERENTIAL DIAGNOSIS OF CHEST PAIN

Chest pain is one of the most common presenting complaints seen by cardiologists. It is important to remember that:

- there are many causes of chest pain
- some causes of chest pain are life-threatening and require prompt diagnosis and treatment; other causes are more benign.

The first differentiation to be made is between cardiac and non-cardiac chest pain (Fig 1.1).

HISTORY TO FOCUS ON THE DIFFERENTIAL DIAGNOSIS OF CHEST PAIN

The differential diagnosis of chest pain is very diverse; a thorough history is, therefore, very important.

PRESENTING COMPLAINT

Differentiation depends on a detailed history of the pain, with particular emphasis on the following characteristics of the pain (Fig. 1.2):

- Whether the pain is continuous or intermittent
- Duration of the pain

- Position of the pain – central or lateral/posterior
- Exacerbating factors – exertion, emotion, food, posture, movement, breathing
- Radiation of the pain – to neck, arms, head
- Quality of pain – crushing, burning, stabbing.

To get an idea of the severity of a patient's symptoms ask them about their 'effort tolerance' – how far can they walk on the flat? Do they have stairs at home, and does walking up them cause chest pain?

Past medical history

This can provide important clues:

- A history of ischaemic heart disease
- A history of peptic ulcer disease, or of frequent ingestion of non-steroidal anti-inflammatory drugs
- Recent operations – cardiothoracic surgery can be complicated by Dressler's syndrome, mediastinitis, ischaemic heart disease or pulmonary embolus (PE)
- Pericarditis might be preceded by a prodromal viral illness
- PE can be preceded by a period of inactivity (e.g. a recent operation, illness or long journey)

Fig. 1.1 Differential diagnosis of chest pain

System involved	Pathology
Cardiac	Myocardial infarction Angina pectoris Pericarditis Prolapse of the mitral valve
Vascular	Aortic dissection
Respiratory (all tend to give rise to pleuritic pain)	Pulmonary embolus Pneumonia Pneumothorax Pulmonary neoplasm
Gastrointestinal	Oesophagitis due to gastric reflux Oesophageal tear Peptic ulcer Biliary disease
Musculoskeletal	Cervical nerve root compression by cervical disc Costochondritis Fractured rib
Neurological	Herpes zoster

- Hypertension is a risk factor for both ischaemic heart disease and dissection of the thoracic aorta.

Drug history, family history and social history

Other risk factors for ischaemic heart disease, such as a positive family history and smoking, should be excluded. A history of heavy alcohol intake is a risk factor for gastritis and peptic ulcer disease.

When a patient presents as a hospital emergency with cardiac chest pain, try to differentiate diagnoses for which thrombolysis is contraindicated from those for which it is indicated. Thrombolysis is contraindicated in pericarditis and dissection of the thoracic aorta.

EXAMINATION OF PATIENTS WHO HAVE CHEST PAIN

Points to note on examination of the patient who has chest pain are shown in Fig. 1.3.

Inspection

On inspection, look for:

- signs of shock (e.g. pallor, sweating) – may indicate myocardial infarction (MI), dissecting aorta, PE
- laboured breathing – may indicate MI leading to left ventricular failure (LVF) or a pulmonary cause
- signs of vomiting – suggests MI or an oesophageal cause
- coughing – suggests LVF, pneumonia.

Cardiovascular system

Note the following:

- Pulse and blood pressure – is there any abnormal rhythm, tachycardia, bradycardia, hypotension, hypertension? Inequalities in the pulses or blood pressure between different extremities are seen in aortic dissection.
- Mucous membranes – pallor could suggest angina due to anaemia; cyanosis suggests hypoxia.
- Any increase in jugular venous pressure – a sign of right ventricular infarction or pulmonary embolus.
- Carotid pulse waveform – a collapsing pulse is seen with aortic regurgitation, which can complicate aortic dissection. It is slow rising if angina is due to aortic stenosis.
- Displaced apex beat, abnormal cardiac impulses (e.g. paradoxical movement in anterior MI).
- Auscultation – listen for a pericardial rub, third heart sound (a feature of LVF), mitral or aortic regurgitation (features of MI or dissection respectively), aortic stenosis (causes angina).

Respiratory system

Note the following signs:

- Breathlessness or cyanosis
- Unequal hemithorax expansion – a sign of pneumonia and pneumothorax
- Abnormal dullness over lung fields – a sign of pneumonia

Fig. 1.2 Characteristics of different types of chest pain

Characteristic	Myocardial ischaemia	Pericarditis	Pleuritic pain	Gastrointestinal pain	Musculoskeletal	Aortic dissection
Quality of pain	Crushing, tight or bandlike	Sharp (may be crushing)	Sharp	Burning	Usually sharp, although can be a dull ache	Sharp, stabbing, tearing
Site of pain	Central anterior chest	Central anterior	Anywhere (usually very localized pain)	Central	Can be anywhere	Retrosternal, interscapular
Radiation	To throat, jaw or arms	Usually no radiation	Usually no radiation	To throat	To arms or around chest to back	Usually no radiation
Exacerbating and relieving factors	Exacerbated by exertion, anxiety, cold; relieved by rest and by glyceryl trinitrate	Exacerbated when lying back; relieved by sitting forward	Exacerbated by breathing, coughing or moving; relieved when breathing stops	Peptic ulcer pain often relieved by food and antacids; cholecystitis and oesophageal pain are exacerbated by food	Can be exacerbated by pressing on chest wall or moving neck	Constant with no exacerbating or relieving factors
Associated features	Patient often sweaty, breathless and shocked; might feel nauseated	Fever, recent viral illness (e.g. rash, arthralgia)	Cough, haemoptysis, breathlessness; shock with pulmonary embolus	Excessive wind	Other affected joints; patient otherwise looks very well	Unequal radial and femoral pulse and blood pressure; aortic regurgitant murmur may be heard on auscultation

- Any bronchial breathing or pleural rub – signs of pneumonia and pleurisy.

Gastrointestinal system

Specifically look for:

- abdominal tenderness or guarding
- scanty or absent bowel sounds – suggests an ileus (e.g. due to perforated peptic ulcer and peritonitis).

INVESTIGATION OF PATIENTS WHO HAVE CHEST PAIN

A summary of tests used to investigate chest pain is shown in Fig. 1.4; an algorithm is given in Fig. 1.5.

Blood tests

These include:

- cardiac biomarkers including cardiac troponin and creatine kinase – cardiac troponin T and I are now commonly used to risk stratify patients presenting with acute coronary syndrome (Fig. 1.6)
- full blood count – anaemia may exacerbate angina
- renal function and electrolytes – may be abnormal if the patient has been vomiting, leading to dehydration and hypokalaemia, or due to diuretic therapy
- arterial blood gases – hypoxia is a sign of PE and LVF, hypocapnoea is seen with hyperventilation
- liver function tests and serum amylase – deranged in cholecystitis and peptic ulcer disease.

5

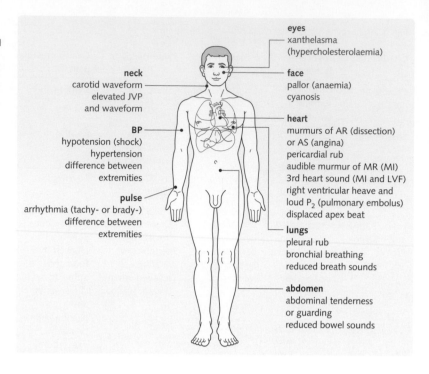

Fig. 1.3 Points to note when examining a patient who has chest pain. AR, aortic regurgitation; AS, aortic stenosis; BP, blood pressure; JVP, jugular venous pressure; LVF, left ventricular failure; MI, myocardial infarction; MR, mitral regurgitation; P2, pulmonary component of the second heart sound.

neck
carotid waveform
elevated JVP and waveform

BP
hypotension (shock)
hypertension
difference between extremities

pulse
arrhythmia (tachy- or brady-)
difference between extremities

eyes
xanthelasma (hypercholesterolaemia)

face
pallor (anaemia)
cyanosis

heart
murmurs of AR (dissection) or AS (angina)
pericardial rub
audible murmur of MR (MI)
3rd heart sound (MI and LVF)
right ventricular heave and loud P_2 (pulmonary embolus)
displaced apex beat

lungs
pleural rub
bronchial breathing
reduced breath sounds

abdomen
abdominal tenderness or guarding
reduced bowel sounds

Fig. 1.4 First-line tests to exclude a chest pain emergency

Test	Diagnosis
ECG	If normal excludes MI, although evidence for this may emerge upon observation
CXR	Widened mediastinum suggests aortic dissection; may show pleural effusion or pulmonary consolidation
Biochemical markers	May be normal in first 4 h after MI, but CK-MB, cardiac troponins will then increase
Arterial blood gases	In the dyspnoeic patient severe hypoxaemia suggests pulmonary embolus, LVF or pneumonia
CT scan	Carry out urgently for suspected aortic dissection

CK-MB, creatine kinase composed of M (muscle) and B (brain) subunits, which is found primarily in cardiac muscle; CT, computed tomography; CXR, chest radiography; ECG, electrocardiography; LVF, left ventricular failure; MI, myocardial infraction.

Electrocardiography

Findings may include:

- ST elevation in absence of bundle branch block (BBB) – indicates acute MI (occasionally it is due to Prinzmetal's angina)

- ST depression in absence of BBB – indicates myocardial ischaemia. At rest this equates with unstable angina or non-Q wave infarction; on exertion this equates with effort-induced angina pectoris or tachyarrhythmias
- BBB – if new this may be due to MI; if it is old, MI cannot be diagnosed from the electrocardiogram (ECG)
- fully developed Q waves – indicate old MI (i.e. over 24-h old)
- atrial fibrillation secondary to any pulmonary disease or myocardial ischaemia.

In the event of a large PE the classic changes are:

- sinus tachycardia (or atrial fibrillation)
- tall P waves in lead II (right atrial dilatation)
- right axis deviation and right BBB
- S wave in lead I, Q wave in lead III, and inverted T wave in lead III (SI QIII TIII pattern seen only with very large PE).

Chest radiography

The following signs may be seen:

- Cardiomegaly
- Widening of the mediastinum in aortic dissection

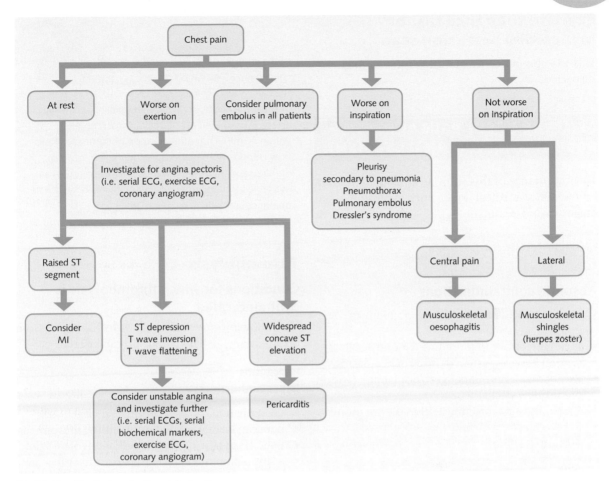

Fig. 1.5 Algorithm for investigation of chest pain.

Fig. 1.6 Cardiac troponin		
	Troponin T level	5-month mortality (FRISC I)
Low risk	<0.06 μg/l	4.3%
Medium risk	0.06–0.18	10.5%
High risk	>0.18	16.1%

- Lung lesions
- Pleural and pericardial effusions
- Oligaemic lung fields in PE.

Echocardiography

This may reveal:

- pericardial effusion – suggests pericarditis or dissection

- regional myocardial dysfunction – a feature of MI or ischaemia
- aortic dissection with false lumen
- aortic or mitral valve abnormalities.

Computed tomography and magnetic resonance imaging

These are the most sensitive methods for excluding aortic dissection and should be performed urgently if this diagnosis is suspected.

It is sometimes possible to visualize PE with spiral computed tomography (CT).

Ventilation/perfusion scan

This excludes PE in most cases if performed promptly. If the V/Q scan is negative and PE is strongly suspected, a more sensitive test is a pulmonary angiogram.

Exercise tolerance test or myocardial perfusion scan

This may be performed at a later date if angina is suspected.

CENTRAL CHEST PAIN AT REST OF RECENT ONSET IN AN ILL PATIENT

The importance of this subject is that this situation represents a medical emergency requiring rapid diagnosis and treatment.

Contraindications to fibrinolytic therapy

Absolute contraindications

- Haemorrhagic stroke or stroke of unknown origin at any time
- Ischaemic stroke in preceding 6 months
- Central nervous system damage or neoplasms
- Recent major trauma/surgery/head injury (within preceding 3 weeks)
- Gastrointestinal bleeding within the last month
- Known bleeding disorder
- Aortic dissection.

Relative contraindications

- Transient ischaemic attack in preceding 6 months
- Oral anticoagulant therapy
- Pregnancy or within 1 week postpartum
- Non-compressible punctures
- Traumatic resuscitation
- Refractory hypertension (systolic blood pressure >180 mmHg)
- Advanced liver disease
- Infective endocarditis
- Active peptic ulcer.

It is necessary in this situation to distinguish between the following:

- MI (see Ch. 10)
- Unstable angina (see Ch. 9)
- Pericarditis (see Ch. 17)
- Dissection of thoracic aorta
- PE
- Mediastinitis secondary to oesophageal tear
- Non-cardiac chest pain.

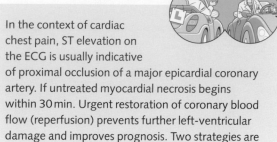

In the context of cardiac chest pain, ST elevation on the ECG is usually indicative of proximal occlusion of a major epicardial coronary artery. If untreated myocardial necrosis begins within 30 min. Urgent restoration of coronary blood flow (reperfusion) prevents further left-ventricular damage and improves prognosis. Two strategies are available: primary angioplasty and thrombolysis. The management will be discussed in Chapter 10.

Thrombolysis

Conditions for which thrombolysis is contraindicated

The following guidelines help differentiate MI from disorders in which thrombolysis can be fatal.

Pericarditis
In pericarditis:

- the patient may have a prodromal viral illness
- pain can be exacerbated by breathing movements
- there might be concomitant indications of infection.
- examination might reveal a pericardial rub – an added sound (or sounds) in the cardiac area on auscultation. This has a scratchy quality and seems close to the ears. If complicated by pericardial effusion, there could be an:
  - impalpable cardiac impulse
  - increased cardiothoracic ratio on the chest radiograph, with a globular heart shadow
- the ECG shows characteristic concave – upwards raised ST segments in all leads except AVR. Thrombolysis is contraindicated because it causes haemopericardium.

Dissection of the thoracic aorta
The pain is sharp and tearing. There is often radiation of the pain to the back. There might be a previous history of hypertension.

On examination, the patient might be shocked and there could be delays between the major pulses (e.g. right brachial versus left brachial, brachial versus femoral).

Chest radiography might show a widened mediastinum. The ECG will not show ST elevation unless the coronary ostia are dissected. Confirmation might require high-resolution spiral CT, echocardiography, or magnetic resonance imaging (which is the best investigation when available; Fig. 1.7).

Thrombolysis is contraindicated because it causes massive bleeding from the aorta (Fig. 1.8).

Mediastinitis

This is unusual and need not usually be considered unless there is a possibility of an oesophageal leak (e.g. after endoscopy or oesophageal surgery).

Pulmonary embolus

Pulmonary emboli can present as acute chest pain in an ill patient or as intermittent chest pain in a relatively well patient. For this reason it is crucial to suspect PE in all patients who have chest pain that is not typically anginal.

The pain of a PE can be pleuritic or tight in nature and might be located anywhere in the chest. It can be accompanied by the following symptoms and signs:

Fig. 1.7 Overview of dissection of the thoracic aorta

Predisposing factors	Hypertension
	Bicuspid aortic valve Pregnancy Marfan's, Turner's, Noonan's syndromes Connective tissue diseases – SLE, Ehlers–Danlos syndrome Men > women Middle age
Pathophysiology	Damage to the media and high intraluminal pressure causing an intimal tear Blood enters and dissects the luminal plane of the media creating a false lumen
Classification	Stanford classification: type A – all dissections involving the ascending aorta; type B – all dissections not involving the ascending aorta
Symptoms	Central tearing chest pain radiating to the back Further complications as the dissection involves branches of the aorta: coronary ostia – myocardial infarction; carotid or spinal arteries – hemiplegia, dysphasia, or paraplegia; mesenteric arteries – abdominal pain
Signs	Shocked, cyanosed, sweating Blood pressure and pulses differ between extremities Aortic regurgitation Cardiac tamponade Cardiac failure
Investigation	CXR – widened mediastinum ± fluid in costophrenic angle ECG – may be ST elevation CT/MRI – best investigations, show aortic false lumen Transoesophageal echo if available is also very sensitive Echocardiography – may show pericardial effusion if dissection extends proximally; tamponade may occur
Management	Pain relief – diamorphine Intravenous access – central and arterial line Fluid replacement – initially colloid then blood when available – crossmatch at least 10 units Blood pressure control – intravenous nitroprusside infusion or labetalol infusion if no cardiac failure – keep blood pressure 120/80 mmHg Surgery for all type A dissections Medical management and possibly surgery or percutaneous treatment for type B

CT, computed tomography; CXR, chest radiography; ECG, electrocardiography; MRI, magnetic resonance imaging; SLE, systemic lupus erythematosus.

Fig. 1.8 Classification of aortic dissections.

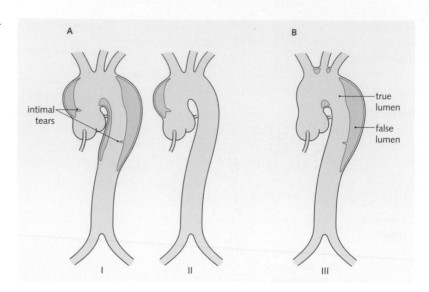

- Dyspnoea
- Dry cough or haemoptysis
- Hypotension and sweating
- Sudden collapse with syncope.

Massive PE will cause collapse with cardiac arrest. The ECG will show ventricular tachyarrhythmias or sinus rhythm with electromechanical dissociation. Patients will often experience a sense of 'impending doom' or profound anxiety.

Conditions predisposing to clot formation in the deep veins of the leg are associated with a high incidence of PE (Fig. 1.9).

As the mortality rate resulting from PE is approximately 10%, appropriate investigations to exclude PE should be carried out promptly and anticoagulation commenced using either intravenous heparin as an infusion or an appropriate low-molecular-weight heparin preparation subcutaneously. Warfarin therapy should be commenced if PE is confirmed.

Fig. 1.9 Conditions predisposing to deep venous thrombosis

Condition	Examples
Immobility	Prolonged bed rest for any reason, long air journeys
Postoperative	Abdominal and pelvic surgery, leg and hip surgery
Haemoconcentration	Diuretic therapy, polycythaemia
Hypercoagulable states	Malignancy, oral contraceptive pill, protein C/protein S deficiency, etc.
Venous stasis (poor flow of venous blood)	Congestive cardiac failure, atrial fibrillation (formation of thrombus in the right ventricle can result in PE)

Dyspnoea

Objectives

By the end of this chapter you should:

- be able to take a history and examine a patient presenting with breathlessness
- understand the appropriate investigations for a patient presenting with breathlessness
- understand the differential diagnosis of a patient presenting with breathlessness.

Dyspnoea is an uncomfortable awareness of one's own breathing. It is considered abnormal only when it occurs at a level of physical activity not normally expected to cause any problem.

DIFFERENTIAL DIAGNOSIS OF DYSPNOEA

Dyspnoea is the main symptom of many cardiac and pulmonary diseases. A working knowledge of the differential diagnosis is required to be able to differentiate acute life-threatening conditions from those that do not require immediate treatment (Fig. 2.1)

HISTORY TO FOCUS ON THE DIFFERENTIAL DIAGNOSIS OF DYSPNOEA

Differentiation depends upon a detailed history of the dyspnoea (Fig. 2.2) with particular emphasis on whether:

- the dyspnoea is acute or chronic
- it is continuous or intermittent
- there are exacerbating and relieving factors – such as exertion, lying flat (suggests orthopnoea in pulmonary oedema), sleep (suggests paroxysmal nocturnal dyspnoea (PND), i.e. waking from sleep gasping for breath in left ventricular failure (LVF))
- there are associated features, such as cough – ask for details of sputum production. Yellow-green

sputum suggests pneumonia or exacerbation of chronic obstructive pulmonary disease (COPD); pink frothy sputum suggests LVF; haemoptysis can be a feature of pneumonia, pulmonary embolism (PE) and carcinoma of the lung

- there is chest pain – ask for details of location, nature of pain, radiation, etc. (see Ch 1)
- there are palpitations – ask about rate and rhythm
- there is ankle oedema – suggestive of congestive cardiac failure, swelling usually worse at the end of the day and best first thing in the morning
- there is a wheeze – suggestive of airways obstruction (i.e. asthma, COPD, or neoplasm of the lung causing airway obstruction). Wheeze can also occur during LVF.

In the investigation of patients with breathlessness it is important to exclude a cardiac source of their symptoms. These include valvular heart disease and left ventricular failure (LVF) – both may be detected by echocardiography. Some patients may have breathlessness as their only symptom of ischaemic heart disease, this is called 'angina equivalent'.

EXAMINATION OF DYSPNOEIC PATIENTS

A thorough examination will be needed because the differential diagnosis is potentially wide (Fig. 2.3).

Fig. 2.1 Differential diagnosis of dyspnoea

System involved	Pathology
Cardiac	Cardiac failure Coronary artery disease Valvular heart disease – aortic stenosis, aortic regurgitation, mitral stenosis/regurgitation, pulmonary stenosis Cardiac arrhythmias
Respiratory	Pulmonary embolus Airway obstruction – COPD, asthma Pneumothorax Pulmonary parenchymal disease (e.g. pneumonia, pulmonary fibrosis, lung neoplasm) Pleural effusion Chest wall limitation – myopathy, neuropathy (e.g. Guillain–Barré disease), rib fracture, kyphoscoliosis
Other	Obesity limiting chest wall movement Anaemia Psychogenic hyperventilation Acidosis (e.g. aspirin overdose, diabetic ketoacidosis)

COPD, *chronic obstructive pulmonary disease.*

Inspection

Note the following:

- Signs of shock, e.g. pallor, sweating – suggest acute LVF, pneumonia, PE
- Inspect for laboured or obstructed breathing (any intercostal recession?), tachypnoea or cyanosis. One or more usually present with resting dyspnoea
- Cough – suggests acute LVF, pneumonia; note the appearance of the sputum (always ask to look in the sputum pot if it is present)
- Appearance of hands and fingers – such as clubbing, carbon dioxide retention flap
- Appearance of chest – a barrel-shaped chest (hyperexpanded) is a feature of emphysema; kyphoscoliosis causes distortion
- Pyrexia – suggests infection (PE or myocardial infarction may be associated with a low-grade pyrexia).

Cardiovascular system

Check the following:

- Pulse and blood pressure – any abnormal rhythm, tachycardia, bradycardia, hypotension, hypertension?
- Mucous membranes – pallor suggests dyspnoea in anaemia; cyanosis suggests hypoxia in LVF, COPD, PE, pneumonia and lung collapse.
- Carotid pulse waveform and jugular venous pressure (JVP) – JVP is elevated in cardiac failure and conditions causing pulmonary hypertension (e.g. PE, COPD).
- Apex beat – displacement suggests cardiac enlargement and a right ventricular heave suggests pulmonary hypertension.
- Heart sounds – note any audible murmurs or added heart sounds (third heart sound in LVF); mitral regurgitation or aortic valve lesions can cause LVF.
- Peripheral oedema.

Respiratory system

Check the following:

- Expansion – unequal thorax expansion is a sign of pneumonia or pneumothorax.
- Vocal fremitus – enhanced vocal fremitus is a sign of consolidation; reduced vocal fremitus is a sign of effusion and pneumothorax.
- Abnormal dullness over hemithorax with reduced expansion – suggests pneumonia.
- Stony dullness at one or both lung bases – suggests pleural effusion.
- Hyperresonance over hemithorax with less expansion – suggests pneumothorax.

Fig. 2.2 Presenting history for different diseases causing dyspnoea

	Cardiac failure	Coronary artery disease	Pulmonary embolus	Pneumothorax	COPD and asthma
Acute or chronic	May be acute or chronic	Acute	Acute (less commonly recurrent small PEs may present as chronic dyspnoea)	Acute	Acute or chronic
Continuous or intermittent	May be continuous or intermittent	Usually intermittent, but an acute MI may lead to continuous and severe LVF	Continuous	Continuous	Continuous or intermittent; these disorders range from the acute, life-threatening exacerbations to chronic, relatively mild episodes
Exacerbating and relieving factors	Exacerbated by exertion and lying flat (orthopnoea and PND may occur) and occasionally by food; relieved by rest, sitting up, oxygen and GTN	Exacerbated by exertion, cold; may be relieved by oxygen			Exacerbated by exertion, pulmonary infections, allergens (e.g. pollen, animal danders); relieved by bronchodilator inhalers
Associated features	May be chest pain (ischaemia may cause LVF); palpitations – arrhythmias may precipitate LVF; cough with pink frothy sputum	Chest pain (central crushing pain radiating to the left arm or throat) and sweating; occasionally palpitations – atrial fibrillation may be precipitated by ischaemia	Pleuritic chest pain (sharp, localized pain worse on breathing and coughing) and bright red haemoptysis; atrial fibrillation may occur	Pleuritic chest pain; there may be a history of chest trauma	Cough with sputum; pleuritic chest pain if associated infection; wheeze

COPD, chronic obstructive pulmonary disease; GTN, glyceryl trinitrate; LVF, left ventricular failure; MI, myocardial infarction; PE, pulmonary embolus; PND, paroxysmal nocturnal dyspnoea.

- Bilateral hyperresonance with loss of cardiac dullness – suggests emphysema.
- Bronchial breathing – suggests pneumonia.
- Crepitations – suggests pneumonia, pulmonary oedema, pulmonary fibrosis.
- Wheeze – asthma, COPD, cardiac asthma in LVF.
- Peak flow test – this is part of every examination of the respiratory system and you should always ask to do this. Explain the technique to the patient clearly and then perform three attempts and take the best out of three. Peak flow will be reduced in active asthma and COPD.

Gastrointestinal system

Examine for hepatomegaly and ascites – seen in congestive cardiac failure or isolated right-sided failure.

INVESTIGATION OF DYSPNOEIC PATIENTS

Algorithms for the diagnosis of acute and chronic dyspnoea are given in Figs 2.4 and 2.5.

Fig. 2.3 Points to note when examining a dyspnoeic patient. BP, blood pressure; CCF, congestive cardiac failure; JVP, jugular venous pressure.

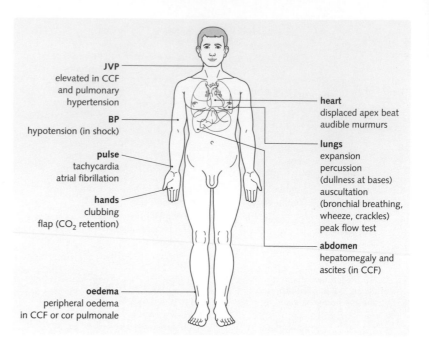

JVP
elevated in CCF
and pulmonary
hypertension

BP
hypotension (in shock)

pulse
tachycardia
atrial fibrillation

hands
clubbing
flap (CO_2 retention)

oedema
peripheral oedema
in CCF or cor pulmonale

heart
displaced apex beat
audible murmurs

lungs
expansion
percussion
(dullness at bases)
auscultation
(bronchial breathing,
wheeze, crackles)
peak flow test

abdomen
hepatomegaly and
ascites (in CCF)

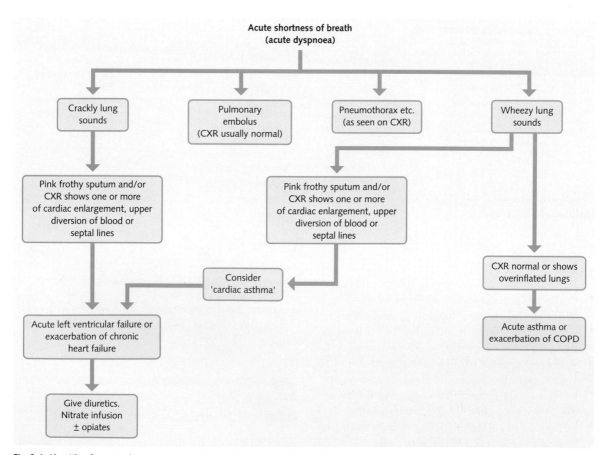

**Acute shortness of breath
(acute dyspnoea)**

Crackly lung
sounds

Pulmonary
embolus
(CXR usually normal)

Pneumothorax etc.
(as seen on CXR)

Wheezy lung
sounds

Pink frothy sputum and/or
CXR shows one or more
of cardiac enlargement, upper
diversion of blood or
septal lines

Pink frothy sputum and/or
CXR shows one or more
of cardiac enlargement, upper
diversion of blood or
septal lines

CXR normal or shows
overinflated lungs

Consider
'cardiac asthma'

Acute left ventricular failure or
exacerbation of chronic
heart failure

Acute asthma or
exacerbation of COPD

Give diuretics.
Nitrate infusion
± opiates

Fig. 2.4 Algorithm for acute dyspnoea. COPD, chronic obstructive pulmonary disease; CXR, chest X-ray; ENT, ear, nose and throat.

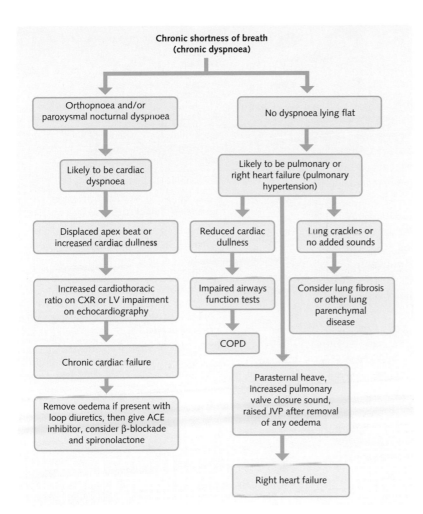

Fig. 2.5 Algorithm for chronic dyspnoea. ACE, angiotensin-converting enzyme; COPD, chronic obstructive pulmonary disease; CXR, chest X-ray; JVP, jugular venous pressure; LV, left ventricle.

A summary of first-line tests to exclude emergencies is shown in Fig. 2.6.

Blood tests

These include:

- Full blood count – might reveal anaemia or leucocytosis (in pneumonia).
- Urea and electrolytes – deranged due to diuretic treatment of cardiac failure, possible syndrome of inappropriate antidiuretic hormone secretion in pneumonia.
- Cardiac enzymes – elevated if dyspnoea secondary to myocardial infarction.
- Liver function tests – deranged in hepatic congestion secondary to congestive cardiac failure.
- Arterial blood gases (Fig. 2.7).

Electrocardiography

This might show:

- ischaemic changes may be seen in patients with coronary artery disease
- sinus tachycardia with SI, QIII, TIII in patients who have had a large PE
- atrial fibrillation – may be seen secondary to any lung pathology or ischaemia.

Chest radiography

Note the following:

- Cardiomegaly in cardiac failure – pulmonary oedema may also be seen (Fig. 2.8).
- Focal lung consolidation in pneumonia (shadowing of a lung segment with an air bronchogram).

Notes on blood gases:

- Hypoxia and hypocapnoea are seen in LVF and pulmonary embolus (this shows a drop in PCO_2 due to hyperventilation as a response to hypoxia).
- Hypoxia and hypercapnoea can occur in COPD and severe asthma – in the former condition this is because the respiratory centre has readjusted to the chronic.
- Hypoxia and oxygen therapy causes the blood PO_2 to rise and the respiratory drive to fall, so ventilation is reduced and the blood PCO_2 rises. In asthma, exhaustion causes the ventilatory drive to fall off and the PCO_2 to rise; this precedes respiratory arrest and is an indication for artificial ventilation of the patient.
- Arterial pH – in acute conditions, such as acute LVF, pulmonary embolus, pneumothorax and early asthma – a respiratory alkalosis occurs (i.e. a low PCO_2 and a high pH of 7.4). The kidneys have not yet compensated by excreting bicarbonate.
- COPD with chronic CO_2 retention – the pH is normal because metabolic compensation has occurred and bicarbonate levels rise as a result of renal retention of bicarbonate (this takes a few days to occur).
- Severe asthma with acute CO_2 retention – the pH falls as the PCO_2 rises as there has been insufficient time for metabolic compensation to occur.

- Pleural effusion – suggests PE, infection or cardiac failure.
- Hyperexpanded lung fields in emphysema (ability to count more than six rib spaces over the lung fields); bullae may be seen in emphysema.
- Presence of a pneumothorax – ask for a film in full expiration if this is suspected.
- Oligaemic lung fields in PE.

Echocardiography

This may reveal:

- LVF
- valve lesions
- left atrial myxoma
- right ventricular hypertrophy and pulmonary hypertension.

Fig. 2.6 First-line tests to exclude a dyspnoeic emergency

Test	Diagnosis
CXR	Acute LVF – pulmonary oedema ± large heart shadow
	Acute asthma – clear overexpanded lungs
	Pneumothorax – absence of lung markings between lung edge and chest wall
	Pneumonia – consolidation
ECG	Look for evidence of MI, ischaemia, pulmonary embolus
Arterial blood gases	Hypoxia suggests LVF or significant lung disease (use the level of hypoxia to guide the need for oxygen therapy or artificial ventilation)
Peak flow	Reduced in airway obstruction (asthma, COPD), but may also be reduced in sick patients because of weakness (it is an effort-dependent test)

COPD, chronic obstructive pulmonary disease; CXR, chest radiography; ECG, electrocardiography; LVF, left ventricular failure; MI, myocardial infarction.

Fig. 2.7 Examples of arterial blood gas results in dyspnoeic patients. The low pH in ventilatory failure is secondary to an acute retention of carbon dioxide. The high pH in acute hyperventilation results from an acute loss of carbon dioxide (respiratory alkalosis). The case of hypoxia shown here has led to hyperventilation and a fall of carbon dioxide and must have been present for some time because the pH is compensated to normal by renal excretion of bicarbonate

	PO_2 (kPa)	PCO_2 (kPa)	pH
Normal range	10.5–13.5	5.0–6.0	7.36–7.44
Ventilatory failure (e.g. chronic obstructive airways disease, severe asthma with exhaustion)	7.0	9.0	7.30
Acute hyperventilation	13.0	4.0	7.48
Hypoxia (e.g. left ventricular failure, pulmonary embolus)	7.5	4.0	7.41

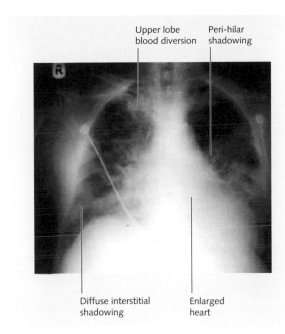

Upper lobe
blood diversion

Peri-hilar
shadowing

Diffuse interstitial
shadowing

Enlarged
heart

Fig. 2.8 Chest X-ray with features of pulmonary oedema.

Ventilation/perfusion scan

This can be used to exclude PE – a mismatched defect with good ventilation and no perfusion is diagnostic of a PE; matched defects are due to infection or COPD or pulmonary scar tissue.

If the ventilation/perfusion (V/Q) scan is negative or equivocal in a high-risk patient, then it might be necessary to consider a contrast-enhanced, high-resolution CT scan as a more sensitive test for PE.

Computed tomography

This is used to obtain detailed visualization of pulmonary fibrosis or small peripheral tumours that cannot be reached with a bronchoscope.

Pulmonary function tests

These tests are used to investigate:

- lung volumes – increased in COPD, reduced in restrictive lung disease
- flow-volume loop – scalloped in COPD
- carbon monoxide transfer – reduced in the presence of normal airway function in restrictive lung diseases.

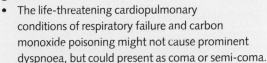

Notes on dyspnoea and arterial blood gases:
- The life-threatening cardiopulmonary conditions of respiratory failure and carbon monoxide poisoning might not cause prominent dyspnoea, but could present as coma or semi-coma.
- Severe hypoxia or tissue underperfusion causes metabolic acidosis (low pH) with normal or low PCO_2.
- Most importantly, arterial blood gases must be performed for all dyspnoeic patients at presentation.

DYSPNOEA AT REST OF RECENT ONSET IN AN ILL PATIENT

This situation is important because it represents a cardiopulmonary emergency requiring rapid diagnosis and treatment. It is necessary to distinguish between the following life-threatening causes:

- Tension pneumothorax
- Life-threatening asthma
- Acute LVF
- PE
- Fulminant pneumonia
- Pneumothorax.

Pneumothorax (air in the pleural space) can cause acute or chronic dyspnoea. A number of possible causes all create a connection between the pleural space and the atmosphere (via either the chest wall or the airways):

- Trauma (e.g. a blow to the chest resulting in fracture of the ribs or insertion of a central venous cannula).
- Rupture of bullae on the surface of the lung – this occurs in some otherwise healthy young patients (more commonly in men than in women) or in patients who have emphysema.

Tension pneumothorax can occur if the air continues to accumulate in the pleural cavity, resulting in a progressive increase in pressure and displacement of the mediastinum away from the side of the lesion. This is characterized by the following clinical signs:

- Severe and worsening dyspnoea
- Displaced trachea and apex beat
- Hyperresonance on the affected side with reduced breath sounds and vocal fremitus
- Progressive hypotension due to reduced venous return and therefore reduced filling of the right ventricle
- Eventual collapse and cardiac arrest and possibly electromechanical dissociation.

Treatment should be immediate, with insertion of a needle into the pleural space to allow gas to escape spontaneously from the pleural cavity. A chest drain should then be inserted and connected to an underwater seal.

Acute asthma

This is another medical emergency requiring prompt diagnosis and treatment. Signs suggestive of a severe asthma attack include:

- the patient being unable to talk in full sentences due to dyspnoea
- the patient sitting forwards and using accessory muscles of respiration – prominent diaphragmatic movements and pursing of the lips on expiration
- tachycardia
- peak flow 30% of normal or less
- pulsus paradoxus – a drop in systolic blood pressure of more than 10 mmHg on inspiration
- silent chest due to severe airflow limitation.

Hypercapnoea on blood gas analysis suggests that the patient is becoming exhausted and respiratory arrest could be imminent – this might occur before there is severe hypoxia. The patient should be considered for intubation and artificial ventilation.

Appropriate treatment with intravenous hydrocortisone, oxygen therapy, nebulized bronchodilators and intravenous fluids should be commenced immediately.

Acute left ventricular failure

The detailed management of acute LVF is discussed in more detail in Chapter 15. The patient needs urgent treatment or will die from asphyxiation. Classic signs of LVF can be seen and include:

- severe dyspnoea
- central cyanosis
- patient sits upright
- bilateral basal fine end-respiratory crepitations (in severe LVF the crepitations extend upwards to fill both lung fields)
- hypotension secondary to poor left ventricular output (common)
- blood gases show hypoxia and often hypocapnoea due to hyperventilation. There is usually a metabolic acidosis as a result of poor tissue perfusion.

Treatment includes high-concentration inhaled oxygen via a mask and intravenous diuretic (frusemide) and diamorphine injections.

Pulmonary embolus

This can present in a number of ways, for example:

- severe dyspnoea
- collapse and syncope
- hypotension
- cardiorespiratory arrest (often with electromechanical dissociation or ventricular fibrillation).

If PE is suspected, anticoagulation should be commenced immediately with an intravenous heparin infusion or subcutaneous low-molecular-weight heparin (LMWH).

If the patient is cardiovascularly unstable, suggesting a massive PE, thrombolysis can be administered or emergency pulmonary angiography carried out in an attempt to disrupt the embolus.

Pneumonia

The patient may be pyrexial or even show signs of septic shock (e.g. hypotension, renal failure). Blood gases may reveal hypoxia, which can be extremely severe in pneumonia caused by *Pneumocystis carinii*.

The chest radiograph might show lobar or patchy consolidation. Radiographic changes can be deceptively mild in mycoplasma or legionella infections.

The most common community-acquired organisms are streptococci and atypical organisms such as mycoplasma, so appropriate antibiotic therapy should be commenced immediately after blood (and sputum if possible) cultures have been taken.

Syncope is a loss of consciousness usually due to a reduction in perfusion of the brain.

DIFFERENTIAL DIAGNOSIS OF SYNCOPE

Many conditions can give rise to loss of consciousness – these can be divided into: cardiac, vasovagal, circulatory, cerebrovascular, neurological and metabolic (Fig. 3.1).

HISTORY TO FOCUS ON THE DIFFERENTIAL DIAGNOSIS OF SYNCOPE

The first differentiation to be made is between cardiac and non-cardiac (usually neurological) syncope.

Differentiation depends upon a detailed history of the syncopal episode with particular emphasis on the features outlined below:

• The events preceding the syncope should be elucidated:
   ○ Exertion – can precipitate syncope in hypertrophic cardiomyopathy (HCM) or aortic stenosis
   ○ Pain or anxiety – in vasovagal syncope
   ○ Standing – can precipitate postural hypotension
   ○ Neck movements – aggravate vertebrobasilar attacks
• Speed of onset of syncope might be:

   ○ immediate with no warning – classic presentation of Stokes-Adams attacks
   ○ rapid with warning – preceded either by lightheadedness (vasovagal) or by an aura (epilepsy)
   ○ gradual with warning – hypoglycaemia preceded by lightheadedness, nausea and sweating
• A witness account of the syncope itself; this is very important; indeed, no history is complete without one:
   ○ Patient lies still, breathing regularly – Stokes-Adams attack (a prolonged Stokes-Adams attack can cause epileptiform movements secondary to cerebral hypoxia).
   ○ Patient shakes limbs or has facial twitching, possibly associated with urinary incontinence and tongue biting – epilepsy.
   ○ Patient becomes very pale and grey immediately before collapsing – vasovagal (patients who have cardiac syncope become very pale after collapse before regaining consciousness).
• The recovery of consciousness can also be characteristic. If the patient:
   ○ feels very well soon after episode – a cardiac cause is likely
   ○ feels washed out and nauseated and takes a few minutes to return to normal – the cause is probably vasovagal
   ○ has a neurological deficit – transient cerebral ischaemia (transient ischaemic attack, TIA) or epilepsy is likely
   ○ is very drowsy and falls asleep soon after regaining consciousness – epilepsy is probable.

Fig. 3.1 Differential diagnosis of syncope (see also Fig. 22.3)

System involved	Pathology
Cardiac	Tachyarrhythmia – supraventricular or ventricular
	Bradyarrhythmia – sinus bradycardia, complete or second-degree heart block, sinus arrest
	Stokes–Adams attack – syncope due to transient asystole
	Left ventricular outflow tract obstruction – aortic stenosis, HCM
	Right ventricular outflow tract obstruction – pulmonary stenosis
	Pulmonary hypertension
Vasovagal (simple faint)	After carotid sinus massage and also precipitated by pain, micturition, anxiety; these result in hyperstimulation by the vagus nerve leading to AV node block (and therefore bradycardia, hypotension and syncope)
Vascular	Postural hypotension – usually due to antihypertensive drugs or diuretics; also caused by autonomic neuropathy as in diabetes mellitus
	Pulmonary embolus – may or may not be preceded by chest pain
	Septic shock – severe peripheral vasodilatation results in hypotension
Cerebrovascular	Transient ischaemic attack
	Vertebrobasilar attack
Neurological	Epilepsy
Metabolic	Hypoglycaemia

AV, *atrioventricular*; HCM, *hypertrophic cardiomyopathy*.

Past medical history

As always a thorough history is needed:

- Any cardiac history is important – ischaemia may precipitate arrhythmias.
- A history of stroke or TIA may suggest a cerebrovascular cause.
- Diabetes mellitus may cause autonomic neuropathy and postural hypotension, whereas good control of diabetes mellitus puts the patient at risk of hypoglycaemia.
- A history of head injury may suggest epilepsy secondary to cortical scarring.

Drug history

Important points include the following:

- Antihypertensives and diuretic agents predispose to postural hypotension.
- Class I and class III antiarrhythmics may cause long QT syndrome and predispose to torsades de points – all antiarrhythmic agents may cause bradycardia leading to syncope.
- Some other drugs may also predispose to long QT syndrome.
- Vasodilators precipitate syncope in pulmonary hypertension.

Family history

A family history of sudden death or recurrent syncope may occur in patients who have hypertrophic cardiomyopathy and also in those rare cases of familial long QT syndrome (Romano-Ward and Jervell-Lange-Nielson syndromes).

A few patients who have epilepsy have a family history.

Social history

Note that:

- alcohol excess is a risk factor for withdrawal fits
- smoking is a risk factor for ischaemic heart disease.

EXAMINATION OF PATIENTS WHO PRESENT WITH SYNCOPE

The points to note on examination of the patient who has syncope are summarized in Fig. 3.2 and discussed in turn below. On inspection, look for any:

- neurological deficit suggestive of a cerebrovascular cause
- signs of shock – such as pallor or sweating.

Notes on syncope:

- Cardiovascular syncope is always accompanied by hypotension.
- Syncope with normal blood pressure is likely to have a neurological, cerebrovascular or metabolic cause.
- Stokes-Adams attacks are episodes of syncope due to cardiac rhythm disturbance.
- Fitting while unconscious is not always caused by epilepsy – it can occur in any patient who has cerebral hypoperfusion or a metabolic disorder (e.g. cardiac syncope or syncope secondary to a pulmonary embolus, cerebrovascular event, hypoglycaemia or alcohol withdrawal).

Cardiovascular system

On examination note the following:

- Pulse – any tachy- or bradyarrhythmia and character of pulse (slow rising in aortic stenosis, jerky in HCM).

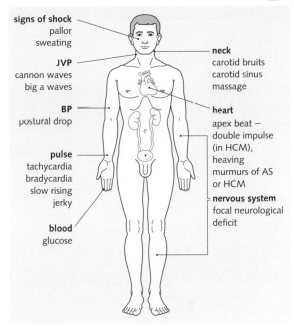

Fig. 3.2 Points to note on examination of a patient presenting with syncope. AS, aortic stenosis; BP, blood pressure; HCM, hypertrophic cardiomyopathy; JVP, jugular venous pressure.

- Blood pressure lying and standing to detect postural hypotension (>20 mmHg drop in blood pressure from lying to standing).
- Jugular venous pulse – cannon waves in complete heart block (due to the atrium contracting against a closed tricuspid valve); prominent 'a' wave in pulmonary hypertension.
- Apex beat – double impulse (HCM), heaving (aortic stenosis).
- Any murmurs.
- Carotid bruits – indicating carotid artery stenosis and cerebrovascular disease.
- Response to carotid sinus massage – apply unilateral firm pressure over the carotid sinus with the patient in bed and attached to a cardiac monitor. Full resuscitative equipment should be easily accessible. Patients who have carotid sinus hypersensitivity will become very bradycardic and may even become asystolic.

Neurological system

This system should be fully examined to detect any residual deficit.

Fingerprick test for blood glucose

This is an easy test and, if positive, may provide valuable diagnostic information.

INVESTIGATION OF PATIENTS WHO PRESENT WITH SYNCOPE

An algorithm for the investigation of syncope is given in Fig. 3.3.

First-line tests to exclude emergencies are shown in Fig. 3.4.

Blood tests

The following tests should be performed:

- Full blood count – anaemia may be secondary to haemorrhage, which will cause postural

hypotension; leucocytosis in sepsis and in the postictal period.
- Electrolytes and renal function – hypokalaemia predisposes towards arrhythmias.
- Calcium – hypocalcaemia is a cause of long QT syndrome.
- Cardiac enzymes – a myocardial infarction may cause sudden arrhythmia.
- Blood glucose.

Electrocardiography

This may show:

- a brady – or tachyarrhythmia
- heart block
- a long QT interval
- ischaemia
- evidence of a pulmonary embolus.

Fig. 3.3 Algorithm for syncope.

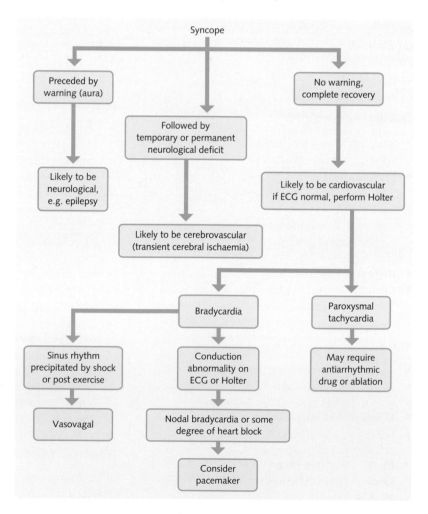

Fig. 3.4 First-line tests to exclude an emergency syncope

Test	Diagnosis
ECG	To look for rhythm disturbance or signs of pulmonary embolus
ECG monitoring on CCU	If suspected cardiac arrhythmia
Temperature, Hb, WBC	To look for septic or haemorrhagic cause
Blood sugar	To look for hypoglycaemia
CT scan	For possible cerebral infarct or TIA, or intracranial bleed causing fits in a patient who has a recent head injury

CCU, coronary care unit; CT, computed tomography; CXR, chest radiography; ECG, electrocardiography; Hb haemoglobin; TIA, transient ischaemic attack; WBC, white blood cell count.

Holter monitor

This is used to provide a 24- or 48-h ECG trace to detect arrhythmias and bradycardias (e.g. sick sinus syndrome, intermittent heart block). Longer cardiac monitoring can be performed using implantable event recorders.

Tilt test

This may aid diagnosis:

- Simple tilt produces hypotension and possibly syncope in autonomic denervation
- Prolonged tilt may provoke vasovagal syncope with bradycardia and hypotension.

Chest radiography

On the chest radiograph:

- there may be cardiomegaly
- the lung fields may be oligaemic due to a PE.

Echocardiography

This may reveal:

- aortic stenosis
- hypertrophic cardiomyopathy
- left atrial enlargement in supraventricular tachycardia
- left atrial thrombus in TIA (transthoracic echocardiography cannot reliably diagnose intracardiac thrombus and if this is suspected as a cause of TIA transoesophageal echocardiography is needed)

- left-ventricular abnormalities in ventricular tachycardia or ventricular fibrillation
- right-ventricular abnormalities in pulmonary hypertension.

Carotid duplex ultrasound scan

This is used to detect carotid atheroma as a source of emboli in TIA. This should be performed regardless of whether carotid bruits are present in a patient who is strongly suspected of having TIAs.

Computed tomography scan of the brain

This may reveal areas of previous infarction in a patient who has had a TIA.

Electrophysiological study of the heart

Consider this if cardiac arrhythmia strongly suspected, but not revealed by Holter monitoring.

Electroencephalography

This will assist in the diagnosis of epilepsy in selected patients.

SYNCOPE OF RECENT ONSET IN AN ILL PATIENT

The importance of this subject is that this situation represents a medical emergency requiring rapid diagnosis and treatment.

It is necessary in this situation to distinguish between the life-threatening causes:

- Intermittent ventricular tachycardia or fibrillation
- Intermittent asystole
- Pulmonary embolus
- Incipient shock
- TIA heralding major stroke
- Hypoglycaemia.

Differentiating features of syncope

The method is to differentiate between cardiac, circulatory and neurological causes.

Cardiac causes

Aortic stenosis

This usually presents as effort-induced syncope because the left ventricular output is restricted by the outflow restriction. The diagnosis is made by feeling a slow rising carotid pulse and a heaving cardiac impulse in the praecordium. An aortic ejection systolic murmur is present. A displaced apex (signifying a dilated ventricle) and signs of heart failure suggest severe aortic stenosis.

Electrocardiography may show left-ventricular hypertrophy. Echocardiography reveals the stenotic valve and assessment by Doppler velocity change through the valve may give an indication of the severity.

A wide variety of ECG abnormalities are possible on a resting ECG. Holter monitoring may reveal an intermittent ventricular arrhythmia. Echocardiography in HCM reveals hypertrophy and subaortic obstruction, and in other cardiomyopathies may reveal a dilated ventricle with poor function. A cardiac electrophysiological study may be necessary in difficult or complex cases.

Tachyarrhythmias

Syncope tends to be due to a supraventricular tachyarrhythmia only if the heart rate is extremely fast. Ventricular tachycardia is more likely to cause syncope because it is accompanied by asynchronous ventricular contraction. If these arrhythmias are not prominent on Holter monitoring, they may be induced during electrophysiological testing.

Bradyarrhythmias

Syncope may occur secondary to a bradyarrhythmia if the cardiac output falls markedly as a consequence of the drop in rate. An ongoing bradyarrhythmia is easily detected on ECG (e.g. sinus bradycardia and second-degree complete heart block). Some conditions, however, occur intermittently and the ECG may be normal after the syncopal episode; for example, heart block may occur intermittently with normal sinus rhythm between episodes.

Ambulatory ECG monitoring is, therefore, needed to capture these episodes. This may be difficult, if they are separated by long periods of time.

Cardiomyopathies

Hypertrophic obstructive cardiomyopathy can give rise to syncope by obstructing left-ventricular outflow on exercise or as a result of ventricular tachycardia or fibrillation. This arrhythmic 'sudden death syndrome'

can also occur in patients who have non-hypertrophic myocardial dysplasias, and patients who have heart failure (dilated cardiomyopathy).

Long QT syndrome

This may be congenital or drug induced, usually by psychiatric or class III antiarrhythmic drugs (see Ch. 11). The syncope is caused by a self-limiting ventricular tachycardia characterized by a systematically rotating QRS vector (torsades de pointes). The tachycardia and syncope are relieved by rapid pacing or pharmacological sinus tachycardia (e.g. using isoprenaline). The resting non-arrhythmic ECG shows QT prolongation.

Circulatory causes

Hypovolaemia

This can present as postural hypotension (i.e. loss of consciousness on standing, relieved by lying flat). This occurs because the blood volume is inadequate, even with an intact baroreflex, to maintain arterial blood pressure in the face of gravity-dependent blood pooling. If this is due to acute haemorrhage there are usually other obvious manifestations such as trauma or haematemesis and melaena. However, internal bleeding can sometimes be difficult to detect. With acute blood loss, the haemoglobin may be normal because there may not have been time for haemodilution to occur.

Septic shock

This causes similar effects by excessive vasodilatation, which prevents baroreflex compensation for postural-dependent blood pooling. However, the patient is usually obviously septic and febrile.

Classic postural hypotension

This is due to inadequate baroreflex control. As well as a drop in blood pressure on standing, there may be very little compensatory tachycardia (part of the baroreflex efferent mechanism is to increase heart rate). This can be formally tested by a simple tilt test, during which there is an excessive blood pressure drop and an inadequate tachycardic response.

Obstruction of pulmonary arteries

Obstruction of pulmonary arteries by embolus enters into the differential diagnosis of all cardiovascular emergencies in which syncope is a feature. Chronic thromboembolism or primary pulmonary hypertension can also lead to postural hypotension because the resistance to right ventricular ejection is too high to allow adequate cardiac output when the filling pressure drops on standing.

Cerebrovascular causes

For full explanation of these syndromes, consult *Crash course: neurology*.

Transient cerebral ischaemia

This often presents to cardiologists because of the known cardiac or arterial causation. These patients show a neurological deficit following the syncope, which recovers with time. There may be repeated episodes. The neurological deficit can often be seen on computed tomography or magnetic resonance scans of the brain. When carotid disease is the source of a cerebral embolus, a bruit may be heard over one or other carotid artery. Even if this is absent, the carotid arteries should be scanned using duplex Doppler to delineate any atheromatous filling defects.

A cardiac source of embolus should be suspected if the patient is in atrial fibrillation.

Left atrial or ventricular thrombus may be difficult to detect by transthoracic echocardiography, in which case a transoesophageal echocardiogram should be performed.

Sometimes TIA is due to an embolus from an infective vegetation of the mitral or aortic valve, or very rarely a left atrial myxoma. These conditions are also investigated by transthoracic and transoesophageal echocardiography.

Patients who have an atrial septal defect may have TIAs secondary to paradoxical emboli (i.e. emboli arising from the right side of the circulation that pass across to the left).

Vertebrobasilar syndrome

This is caused by obstruction of the arteries to the posterior part of the brain (brain stem and cerebellum). The syncope may be preceded by vertigo or dizziness. Precipitation by neck movement is a classical feature in this syndrome when it is associated with cervical spondylosis because the vertebral arteries course within the cervical vertebrae and can get kinked if there is osteoarthritis.

Other neurological causes

Neurological causes without any cardiac or arterial aetiology should be studied in *Crash course: neurology*, but epilepsy should always be borne in mind during history taking.

Metabolic causes

For rare causes see *Crash course: metabolism and nutrition*.

In the common situation of insulin-dependent diabetes mellitus, most patients are inadequately controlled, which leads to more rapid development of heart disease and autonomic neuropathy. Fear of this drives some patients to control their diabetes mellitus very obsessively and tightly. These patients tend to experience episodes of loss of consciousness due to hypoglycaemia. However, hypoglycaemia can occur in any treated diabetic patient and may be precipitated by exercise or a reduction in food intake.

Palpitations

Objectives

By the end of this chapter you should:

- be able to take a history and examine a patient who presents with palpitations
- understand the differential diagnosis of the causes of palpitations
- understand the appropriate investigations for a patient who presents with palpitations.

Palpitations are an unpleasant awareness of the heart beat. They may be rapid, slow or just very forceful beats at a normal rate.

DIFFERENTIAL DIAGNOSIS OF PALPITATIONS

Palpitations may be caused by any disorder producing a change in cardiac rhythm or rate and any disorder causing increased stroke volume.

Rapid palpitations

These may be regular or irregular. Regular palpitations may be a sign of:

- sinus tachycardia
- atrial flutter
- atrial tachycardia
- supraventricular re-entry tachycardia.

  Irregularly irregular palpitations may indicate:

- atrial fibrillation
- multiple atrial or ventricular ectopic beats.

Slow palpitations

Patients often describe these as missed beats or forceful beats (after a pause the next beat is often more forceful due to a long filling time and, therefore, a higher stroke volume). The following may be causes of slow palpitations:

- Sick sinus syndrome
- Atrioventricular block
- Occasional ectopics with compensatory pauses.

Disorders causing increased stroke volume

Increased stroke volume may result from:

- valvular lesions (e.g. mitral or aortic regurgitation)
- high-output states (e.g. pregnancy, thyrotoxicosis or anaemia).

HISTORY TO FOCUS ON THE DIFFERENTIAL DIAGNOSIS OF PALPITATIONS

When taking a history from a patient complaining of palpitations, aim to find answers to the following three questions:

1. What is the nature of the palpitations?
2. How severe or life-threatening are they?
3. What is the likely underlying cause?

Nature of the palpitations

Ask the patient to describe the palpitations by tapping them out (fast, slow, regular or irregular). Are the palpitations continuous or intermittent (paroxysmal is the term used for intermittent tachycardias), is the onset of the palpitations sudden or progressive?

Severity of the palpitations

Determine the severity of the palpitations (i.e. are they associated with complications such as cardiac failure, exacerbation of ischaemic heart disease or thromboembolic events?).

Are the palpitations associated with:

- syncope, dizziness or shortness of breath – suggesting that cardiac output is compromised?
- angina – suggesting they are causing or being caused by underlying ischaemic heart disease?
- a history of stroke or transient ischaemic attack or limb ischaemia – suggesting thromboembolic complications of arrhythmia?

Likely underlying causes of palpitation

Are there any features in the history suggestive of the recognized causes of arrhythmias shown in Fig. 4.1.

EXAMINATION OF PATIENTS WHO HAVE PALPITATIONS

Remember, when examining any patient who has a supposedly cardiac problem you must perform a thorough examination of all systems. Cardiac disease can both cause and be caused by disease in other systems, so don't get caught out.

Fig. 4.2 summarizes the important points in the examination of a patient who has palpitations, which are outlined below.

General observation

Look for:

- cyanosis – suggestive of cardiac failure or lung disease (remember that pulmonary embolus is a well-recognized cause of tachyarrhythmia)
- dyspnoea – suggestive of cardiac failure or lung disease
- pallor – suggestive of anaemia
- thyrotoxic or myxoedematous facies.

Cardiovascular system

Pulse

Note the rate, rhythm and character of the pulse at the radial artery (time it for at least 15 s). Information on the character of the pulse is often more clearly elicited from the carotid pulse, especially features such as a:

- slow rising pulse – due to aortic stenosis
- collapsing pulse – due to aortic regurgitation.

A high-volume pulse (due to high-output states and aortic or mitral regurgitation) is often most easily felt at the radial pulse, where it is felt as an abnormally strong pulsation.

Blood pressure

This may be low if the patient has palpitations. Hypertension is a cause of atrial fibrillation. A wide pulse pressure is a sign of aortic regurgitation.

Jugular venous pressure

The jugular venous pressure may be elevated if the patient has congestive cardiac failure as a consequence of an uncontrolled tachycardia or has atrial flutter or fibrillation secondary to pulmonary embolism.

Fig. 4.1 Features in the history that might suggest the cause of an arrhythmia

Features in the history	Cause of arrhythmia
Chest pain, breathlessness on exertion, history of myocardial infarction, history of bypass surgery	Ischaemic heart disease
Tremor, excessive sweating, unexplained weight loss, lethargy, obesity, history of thyroid surgery	Thyroid disease
History of rheumatic fever	Heart valve disease
Peptic ulcer disease, menorrhagia, recent operation	Anaemia
Alcohol, caffeine, amphetamine, antiarrhythmic agents	Proarrhythmic drugs
Anxiety	Anxiety

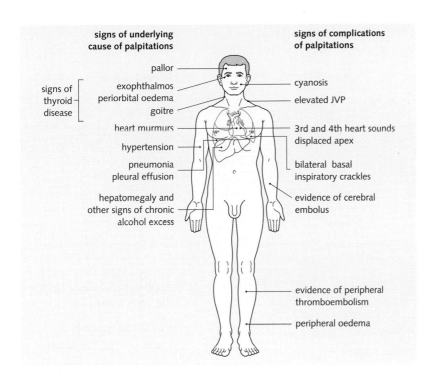

Fig. 4.2 Important points to note when examining a patient who has palpitations. CVA, cerebrovascular accident; JVP, jugular venous pressure.

In the figure:

signs of underlying cause of palpitations

- pallor
- signs of thyroid disease
  - exophthalmos
  - periorbital oedema
  - goitre
- heart murmurs
- hypertension
- pneumonia pleural effusion
- hepatomegaly and other signs of chronic alcohol excess

signs of complications of palpitations

- cyanosis
- elevated JVP
- 3rd and 4th heart sounds displaced apex
- bilateral basal inspiratory crackles
- evidence of cerebral embolus
- evidence of peripheral thromboembolism
- peripheral oedema

Apex beat

This may be displaced in a patient who has left-ventricular failure.

Heart sounds

A third or fourth heart sound may be heard. Murmurs of mitral or aortic regurgitation are possible causes of high-output state. The murmur of mitral stenosis may be heard in patients who have atrial fibrillation.

Respiratory system

Bilateral basal inspiratory crepitations are heard in a patient who has left-ventricular failure. There may be signs of an underlying chest infection (consolidation or effusion), a common cause of palpitations.

Gastrointestinal system

Hepatomegaly and ascites may be signs of congestive cardiac failure or alcoholic liver disease – alcohol is one of the most common causes of tachyarrhythmias. Look for other signs of liver disease if this is suspected.

Limbs

On examining the limbs note the following points:

- Peripheral oedema may be a sign of congestive cardiac failure
- Tremor may be a sign of thyrotoxicosis or alcohol withdrawal
- Brisk reflexes seen in thyrotoxicosis
- Weakness – may be a sign of previous cerebral embolus.

INVESTIGATION OF PATIENTS WHO HAVE PALPITATIONS

An algorithm for the investigation of palpitations is given in Fig. 4.3.

Blood tests

The following blood tests may aid diagnosis:

- Electrolytes – hypokalaemia is an aggravating factor for most tachyarrhythmias
- Full blood count – anaemia or a leucocytosis suggesting sepsis may be evident

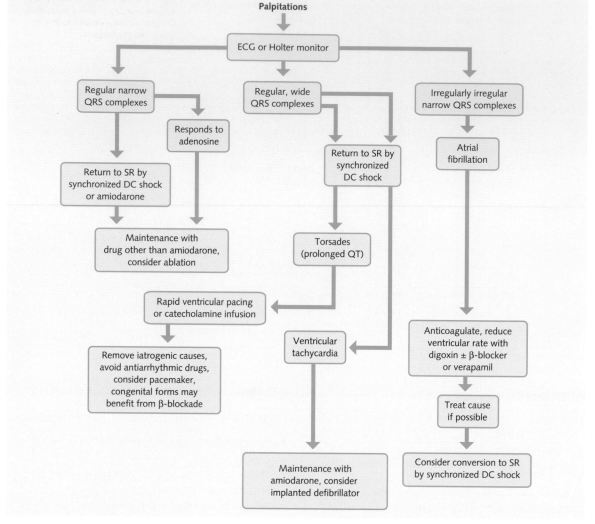

Fig. 4.3 Algorithm for palpitations. SR, sinus rhythm.

- Thyroid function tests
- Liver function tests – deranged in congestive cardiac failure or alcoholic liver disease.

Electrocardiography

12-lead electrocardiography

This may enable the diagnosis to be made instantly. However, if the palpitations are intermittent or paroxysmal the ECG may be normal.

There may be signs of the cause of the palpitations on the ECG, for example ischaemia, hypertension or presence of a delta wave or short PR interval as seen in some congenital causes of paroxysmal tachyarrhythmias, such as Wolff–Parkinson–White syndrome (pre-excitation).

24-h electrocardiography

Monitoring of the ECG for 24 h may reveal paroxysmal arrhythmias. Patients note down the times that palpitations occur and these can be compared with the recorded ECG at that time. Monitors are available that record the ECG for longer periods (e.g. 72-h tape), to diagnose more infrequent episodes.

Exercise electrocardiography

This test can be used to reveal exercise-induced arrhythmias. Examples of ECGs illustrating atrial fibrillation, atrial flutter and supraventricular re-entry tachycardia (SVT) are shown in Fig. 4.4.

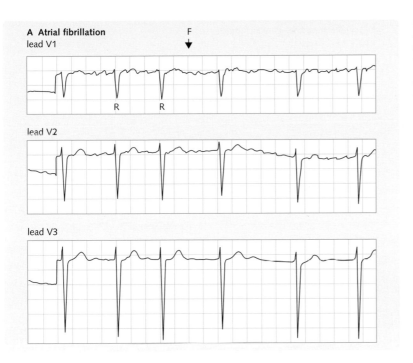

A Atrial fibrillation
lead V1

F

R   R

lead V2

lead V3

Fig. 4.4 Electrocardiograms illustrating atrial fibrillation, atrial flutter and supraventricular re-entry tachycardia. (A) Note the narrow QRS complexes. Fibrillation waves (F) can sometimes be seen. Note the irregularly irregular rhythm and the absence of P waves preceding the QRS complexes. The baseline may show an irregular fibrillating pattern.

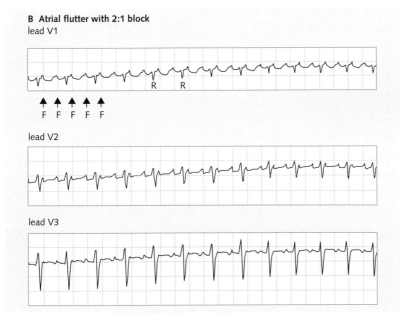

B Atrial flutter with 2:1 block
lead V1

R   R

F F F F F

lead V2

lead V3

Fig. 4.4 (B) Note the regular rhythm with a rate divisible into 300 (150 beats/min in this case). The P waves are seen in all three leads, but best in V1 at a rate of 300/min. Occasionally, the F (flutter) waves form a sawtooth-like pattern (not shown here). Note the F waves at 200-ms intervals (300/min), narrow QRS and regular RR intervals at 400 ms (150/min).

Fig. 4.4 (C) The rhythm is regular and fast (usually 140–240 beats/min). P waves can be seen; these can occur before or after the QRS. Point X shows reversion back to sinus rhythm – note that the following beat has a normal P wave preceding it.

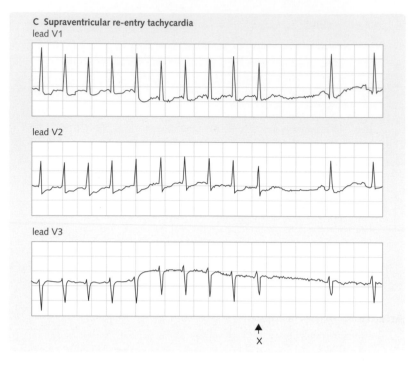

C Supraventricular re-entry tachycardia

lead V1

lead V2

lead V3

X

Vagotonic manoeuvres

Such manoeuvres include:

- Valsalva manoeuvre
- carotid sinus massage
- diving reflex
- painful stimuli.

Vagotonic manoeuvres should be clearly explained to the patient before they are performed – they can be painful and care should be taken. Given the risk of profound bradycardia or asystole patients should always be connected to a cardiac monitor, with i.v. access and resuscitation equipment available.

These manoeuvres all act by increasing vagal tone, which in turn increases the refractory period of the atrioventricular (AV) node and increases AV node conduction time. By doing this it is possible to differentiate between three common tachyarrhythmias that are sometimes indistinguishable on ECG recording:

1. Atrial flutter
2. Atrial fibrillation
3. Supraventricular re-entry tachycardia.

The first thing to do when you see a fast heart rhythm is to establish the clinical status of the patient. Following this, determine if it is narrow complex (atrial flutter, SVT) or broad complex tachycardia (ventricular tachycardia). You also need to determine whether the rhythm is regular (atrial flutter, SVT or VT) or irregular (atrial fibrillation).

Broad complex tachycardia can occur in atrial fibrillation or atrial flutter when there is also aberrant conduction across the AV node. However, any broad complex tachycardia should always be assumed to be of ventricular origin, because it is sometimes difficult to differentiate between them.

Fig. 4.5 Characteristic features of atrial fibrillation, atrial flutter and supraventricular re-entry tachycardia

	Atrial fibrillation	Atrial flutter	Supraventricular re-entry tachycardia
Rate	Any rate; pulse deficit if fast	Atrial flutter rate is 300/min; the ventricular response is therefore divisible into this (usually 100 or 150/min)	140–260 beats/min
Rhythm	Irregularly irregular	Regular	Regular
Response to adenosine or Valsalva manoeuvre	Slowing of ventricular rate reveals underlying lack of P waves	Slowing of ventricular rate reveals underlying flutter waves	Blocking the AV node might 'break' the re-entry circuit and terminate the tachycardia

AV node, atrioventricular node.

The characteristic features of these tachyarrhythmias are listed in Fig. 4.5.

Adenosine administration

Adenosine is a purine nucleoside that acts to block the AV node. When administered intravenously it will achieve complete AV block. Its half-life is very short (only a few seconds), so this effect is very short lived.

Side effects of adenosine include bronchospasm, so avoid in asthmatics.

Chest radiography

Look for:

- evidence of valve disease (e.g. large left atrium and pulmonary vascular congestion in mitral stenosis)
- evidence of cardiac failure – enlarged heart shadow, pulmonary oedema
- Kerley B lines (horizontal lines of fluid-filled fissures at the costophrenic angle)
- evidence of pulmonary disease – effusion, collapse or consolidation.

Echocardiography

This will reveal any valvular pathology. It also enables evaluation of left-ventricular function.

Electrophysiological study

This is useful in investigating patients suspected of having tachyarrhythmias due to abnormal re-entry pathways. The technique enables localization of the re-entry circuit, which may then be ablated using a radiofrequency thermal electrode placed inside the heart.

Other investigations

Various other investigations may be required to identify a suspected cause of the palpitations. These depend upon the clinical evidence, for example:

- V/Q scan, if a pulmonary embolus is likely
- coronary angiogram, if coronary artery disease is suspected.

Whenever investigating, examining or taking a history from a patient with palpitations it is always useful to identify the nature, severity and likely underlying cause of the palpitations. This will help you to structure your approach and to present your findings in a logical manner.

Peripheral oedema

By the end of this chapter you should:

- be able to take a history and examine a patient who presents with peripheral oedema
- understand the causes of peripheral oedema
- understand the appropriate investigations for a patient who presents with peripheral oedema.

Peripheral oedema is caused by an increase in extracellular fluid. The fluid will follow gravity and, therefore, the ankles are the first part affected in the upright patient. Ankle swelling is indicative of oedema if there is not a local acute or chronic traumatic cause. Oedema may be a feature of generalized fluid retention or obstruction of fluid drainage from the lower limbs.

DIFFERENTIAL DIAGNOSIS OF OEDEMA

There are a number of causes of oedema that can be divided into five main groups (Fig. 5.1):

1. Cardiac failure – this is due to increased sodium retention secondary to activation of the renin-angiotensin system.
2. Hypoalbuminaemia – loss of oncotic pressure within the capillaries causes loss of fluid from the intravascular space.
3. Renal impairment – reduction in sodium excretion results in water retention.
4. Hepatic cirrhosis – there are a number of mechanisms involved: hypoalbuminaemia (occurs as the hepatic synthetic activity is reduced), peripheral vasodilatation and activation of the renin-angiotensin system with resulting sodium retention.
5. Drugs (e.g. corticosteroids).

HISTORY TO FOCUS ON THE DIFFERENTIAL DIAGNOSIS OF PERIPHERAL OEDEMA

The first differentiation to be made is between cardiac and non-cardiac oedema. The cause of the oedema is usually revealed by a detailed systems review because there are often symptoms related to the underlying disorder. Associated breathlessness suggests:

- pulmonary oedema – this can occur due to cardiac failure or renal failure
- chronic lung disease (e.g. chronic obstructive airways disease causes breathlessness)
- primary and thromboembolic pulmonary hypertension – cause breathlessness and right heart failure.

Other important signs and symptoms include:

- chest pain and palpitations – suggest underlying cardiac disease (ischaemia or arrhythmias, respectively)
- a history of alcohol or drug abuse or of previous liver disease – suggests a hepatic cause for the oedema
- diarrhoea – may be due to a protein-losing enteropathy.

Past medical history

A detailed history of all previous illnesses and operations will provide clues in a patient who has longstanding cardiac, hepatic or liver disease.

Fig. 5.1 Differential diagnosis of peripheral oedema

Pathology	Cause
Congestive cardiac failure	Myocardial infarction, recurrent tachyarrhythmias (particularly atrial fibrillation), hypertensive heart disease, myocarditis, cardiomyopathy due to drugs and toxins, mitral, aortic, or pulmonary valve disease
Right heart failure secondary to pulmonary hypertension (cor pulmonale)	Chronic lung disease, primary pulmonary hypertension
Hypoalbuminaemia	Excessive protein loss (due to nephrotic syndrome, extensive burns, protein-losing enteropathy), reduced protein production (due to liver failure) or inadequate protein intake (due to protein-energy malnutrition)
Renal disease	Any cause of renal impairment (e.g. hypertension, diabetes mellitus, autoimmune disease, infection)
Liver cirrhosis	Alcohol, hepatitis A, B, C, autoimmune chronic active hepatitis, biliary cirrhosis, Wilsons disease, haemochromatosis, drugs
Idiopathic	Premenstrual oedema
Arteriolar dilatation (exposing the capillaries to high pressure, so increasing intravascular hydrostatic pressure)	Dihydropyridine calcium channel blockers (e.g. nifedipine, amlodipine)
Sodium retention	Cushing's disease resulting in excessive mineralocorticoid activity, corticosteroids

Drug history

Important points include the following:

- Some drugs may be renotoxic (e.g. non-steroidal anti-inflammatory agents, angiotensin-converting enzyme inhibitors).
- Some drugs may be hepatotoxic (e.g. methotrexate).
- Dihydropyridine calcium channel blockers cause ankle oedema in some patients.

Social history

Important findings may include:

- cigarette smoking – a risk factor for ischaemic heart disease

Causes of localized oedema in either the arms or legs include:
- local venous thrombosis or compression
- local cellulitis
- local trauma
- lymphoedema secondary to obstruction of lymphatic drainage (e.g. secondary to malignancy).

- intravenous drug abuse – a risk factor for hepatitis
- alcohol abuse – a risk factor for hepatic cirrhosis.

EXAMINATION OF PATIENTS WHO HAVE OEDEMA

A thorough examination of all systems usually reveals the underlying disease.

Cardiovascular system

Check the pulse and blood pressure:

- The pulse is often fast in the patient who has cardiac failure.
- Blood pressure may be low.
- Patients who have chronic renal disease are often hypertensive.

Check the jugular venous pressure (JVP). This is elevated in all patients who have generalized fluid overload and is, therefore, not a specific sign (only an isolated elevated JVP in the absence of oedema is specific for right-ventricular failure).

On examination of the praecordium:

- the apex may be dyskinetic and laterally displaced in the patient who has cardiac failure
- there may be a left parasternal heave suggestive of right-ventricular strain
- there may be added third and fourth heart sounds in cardiac failure (a 'gallop' rhythm)
- audible murmurs may be present suggesting a valvular cause for cardiac failure.

Respiratory system

On inspection, consider the following:

- The patient may be tachypnoeic and cyanosed – this may be secondary to cardiac or respiratory disease.
- The lungs may be hyperinflated (due to emphysema) or show reduced expansion.

Expansion is reduced in all causes of lung disease, except perhaps primary pulmonary hypertension.

The lung bases may be stony dull (with absent breath sounds) indicating bilateral pleural effusions – these are a sign of generalized fluid retention.

Findings on auscultation of the lungs can include:

- bilateral basal fine inspiratory crepitations suggesting left ventricular failure
- coarse crepitations or wheeze, which may be heard in bronchitis or emphysema
- mid-inspiratory crepitations, which may be heard in pulmonary fibrosis.

Gastrointestinal system

Points to consider on inspection are as follows:

- Does the patient have signs of chronic liver disease, such as jaundice, liver flap, spider naevi, gynaecomastia, loss of pubic hair and testicular atrophy?
- Does the patient have renal failure and look uraemic?

Palpation of the abdomen may reveal ascites in patients who have liver, cardiac or renal disease. A *caput medusae* may be evident.

Renal system

On inspection:

- the patient may have earthy discoloration of the skin secondary to uraemia

- patients with renal failure may be anaemic (pale sclerae)
- there might be evidence of ongoing dialysis, either though the presence of fistulae (usually in the forearms) or tubing attached to the abdomen in ambulatory peritoneal dialysis.

On examination:

- patients are occasionally hypertensive
- the JVP may be raised as a result of fluid retention
- lung bases may be stony dull due to bilateral pleural effusions
- auscultation may reveal a pericardial rub
- bilateral basal inspiratory crepitations suggest pulmonary congestion.

Dipstick the urine – this is part of every examination of the cardiovascular system. Proteinuria is a feature of nephrotic syndrome and other causes of renal impairment. Haematuria is seen in some diseases causing renal impairment.

Examination of the oedema

Oedema of generalized fluid retention is pitting in nature. To demonstrate this, the area in question should be pressed firmly for at least 15 s – there will be an indent in the oedema after this. Be careful: ankle oedema is often tender. The severity of the ankle oedema can be roughly gauged by the extent to which the oedema can be felt up the leg. Lymphoedema and chronic venous oedema do not 'pit'. Fig. 5.2 summarizes the findings in patients who have ankle swelling.

When assessing a patient with peripheral oedema for the first time it is useful to ask about ankle swelling – as fluid follows gravity it is often first noticed in the lower limbs in the mobile patient, and may be most pronounced by the end of the day. In the supine patient this swelling may also be detectable around the sacrum.

INVESTIGATION OF PATIENTS WHO HAVE OEDEMA

An algorithm for the investigation of peripheral oedema is given in Fig. 5.3.

Fig. 5.2 Signs in patients who present with ankle swelling. BP, blood pressure; CCF, congestive cardiac failure; COPD, chronic obstructive pulmonary disease; JVP, jugular venous pressure; LVF, left ventricular failure.

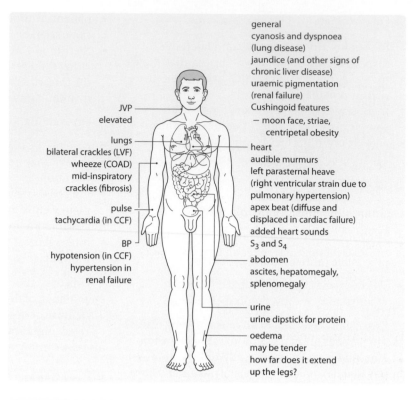

general
cyanosis and dyspnoea
(lung disease)
jaundice (and other signs of chronic liver disease)
uraemic pigmentation
(renal failure)
Cushingoid features
— moon face, striae, centripetal obesity

JVP
elevated

lungs
bilateral crackles (LVF)
wheeze (COAD)
mid-inspiratory crackles (fibrosis)

heart
audible murmurs
left parasternal heave
(right ventricular strain due to pulmonary hypertension)
apex beat (diffuse and displaced in cardiac failure)
added heart sounds
S_3 and S_4

pulse
tachycardia (in CCF)

BP
hypotension (in CCF)
hypertension in renal failure

abdomen
ascites, hepatomegaly, splenomegaly

urine
urine dipstick for protein

oedema
may be tender
how far does it extend up the legs?

Fig. 5.3 Algorithm for peripheral oedema. ACE, angiotensin-converting enzyme; CXR, chest X-ray; JVP, jugular venous pressure; LV, left ventricular.

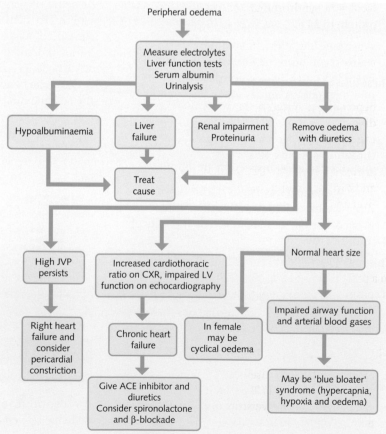

Peripheral oedema

Measure electrolytes
Liver function tests
Serum albumin
Urinalysis

Hypoalbuminaemia

Liver failure

Renal impairment
Proteinuria

Remove oedema with diuretics

Treat cause

High JVP persists

Increased cardiothoracic ratio on CXR, impaired LV function on echocardiography

Normal heart size

Right heart failure and consider pericardial constriction

Chronic heart failure

In female may be cyclical oedema

Impaired airway function and arterial blood gases

Give ACE inhibitor and diuretics
Consider spironolactone and β-blockade

May be 'blue bloater' syndrome (hypercapnia, hypoxia and oedema)

Blood tests

The following blood tests should be considered:

- Full blood count – anaemia is common in chronic renal disease and can precipitate cardiac failure.
- Renal function – this is abnormal in renal disease, but note that patients who have longstanding cardiac or liver disease often have deranged renal function.
- Liver function – this is abnormal in liver disease, but note that hepatic congestion due to cardiac failure also causes abnormal liver function tests.
- Plasma albumin concentration.
- Thyroid function – hyperthyroidism may precipitate cardiac failure, hypothyroidism can cause oedema.

Urine tests

With urine tests, note:

- A 24-h urine protein excretion test is mandatory if there is no evidence of cardiac disease and the plasma albumin is low.
- Nephrotic syndrome causes loss of at least 3 g protein in 24 h.

Arterial blood gases

These tests may aid diagnosis of:

- hypoxia, which may be caused by lung or cardiac disease
- carbon dioxide retention, which is a sign of chronic obstructive airways disease
- acidosis, which can occur with normal oxygen and carbon dioxide (metabolic acidosis) in both liver and renal failure.

Electrocardiography

This may show evidence of old myocardial infarction in a patient who has cardiac failure. Atrial fibrillation is common in patients with heart failure.

Chest radiography

Chest radiography may help diagnose:

- cardiomegaly (increased cardiothoracic ratio)
- pulmonary oedema ('Bats wing shadowing, upper lobe blood diversion, effusions, Kerley B lines)

- pleural effusions
- lung overexpansion.

Echocardiography

This may show impaired ventricular function, and a dilated ventricle. Valve lesions may also be seen.

Ultrasound

Regarding ultrasound:

- in a patient who has no evidence of cardiac, renal or liver disease and bilateral ankle oedema, a venous obstruction or external compression must be excluded
- Doppler ultrasound to detect venous thrombosis and ultrasound of the pelvis to exclude a mass lesion causing compression are appropriate.

IMPORTANT ASPECTS

Salt and water retention

It is important to appreciate that oedema in heart failure is due to generalized salt and water retention, which results from the neurohumoral response to heart failure (see Ch. 15 and Fig. 5.4). The symptoms and signs do not, therefore, differ from those due to generalized salt and water retention in other conditions with similar neurohumoral response. A similar picture is obtained when the salt and water retention is primarily renal in origin.

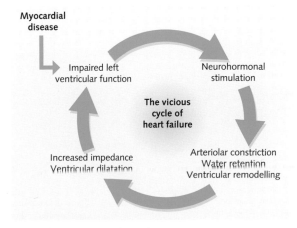

Fig. 5.4 The vicious cycle of heart failure.

Increase in extracellular water and intravascular blood volume

Salt and water retention cause an increase in extracellular water and intravascular blood volume. The increase in volume of blood in the heart and central vessels increases pressures, including right atrial pressure. This is appreciated clinically as raised JVP. It can be observed very simply that the appearance of oedema occurs first and that the increase in JVP follows as the central compartment subsequently fills up. When diuretics are administered, the JVP goes down first before the peripheral oedema disappears. Therefore, it is incorrect to diagnose right heart failure from a raised JVP in the presence of oedema, but only where the JVP is raised when oedema is absent or has been removed.

Hypertension treated with calcium antagonists

Oedema commonly appears in patients who have hypertension treated with the dihydropyridine calcium antagonists (e.g. nifedipine, amlodipine). This is due to disturbance of Starling's forces in the tissue, not to general fluid retention. This type of oedema should not be treated with diuretics, which cause electrolyte depletion.

Heart murmur

Objectives

By the end of this chapter you should:

- be able to take a history and examine a patient with a heart murmur
- understand the differential diagnosis for the causes of a heart murmur
- understand the appropriate investigations for a patient presenting with a heart murmur.

A heart murmur is the sound caused by turbulence of blood flow, which occurs when the velocity of blood is disproportionate to the size of the orifice it is moving through.

DIFFERENTIAL DIAGNOSIS OF A HEART MURMUR

Many conditions can give rise to a murmur:

- Valve lesions – either stenosis or regurgitation of any heart valve
- Left-ventricular outflow obstruction – an example is hypertrophic cardiomyopathy (HCM)
- Ventricular septal defect
- Vascular disorders – coarctation of the aorta, patent ductus arteriosus, arteriovenous malformations (pulmonary or intercostal) and venous hum (cervical or hepatic)
- Increased blood flow – normal anatomy, but increased blood flow as in high-output states. Examples of high-output states are anaemia, pregnancy, thyrotoxicosis or childhood
- Increased flow across a normal pulmonary valve in atrial and ventricular septal defect.

Cardiac sounds can be confused for murmurs. These include:
- third and fourth heart sounds
- mid-systolic clicks, heard in mitral valve prolapse
- pericardial friction rub.

A differential diagnosis of heart murmur is shown in Fig. 6.1.

HISTORY TO FOCUS ON THE DIFFERENTIAL DIAGNOSIS OF A HEART MURMUR

When taking a history from a patient who has a heart murmur, aim to answer the following questions:
- What is the possible aetiology of the murmur e.g. infective endocarditis, valve lesion secondary to rheumatic heart disease, high-output state, etc.?
- Are there any complications of valve disease e.g. cardiac failure, exacerbation of ischaemic heart disease, arrhythmias, syncope, etc.?

Presenting complaint

Common presenting complaints include:

- shortness of breath – suggestive of cardiac failure; also ankle swelling, paroxysmal nocturnal dyspnoea and fatigue
- chest pain – due to ischaemic heart disease or atypical chest pain seen in patients who have mitral valve prolapse
- syncope – especially seen in patients who have left-ventricular outflow obstruction (e.g. aortic stenosis or HCM)
- fever, rigors and malaise – common presenting complaints in patients who have infective endocarditis
- palpitations – for example, mitral valve disease is associated with atrial fibrillation.

Fig. 6.1 Differential diagnosis of heart murmur

Phase of cardiac cycle	Nature of murmur	Valve lesion	Cause of valve lesion
Systolic	Ejection systolic	Aortic stenosis (AS)	Valvular stenosis, congenital valvular abnormality, rheumatic fever, supravalvular stenosis, subvalvular stenosis, senile valvular calcification
		Aortic sclerosis	Aortic valve roughening
		HCM	Left ventricular outflow tract (subaortic) stenosis
		Increased flow across normal valve	High-output states (e.g. anaemia, fever, pregnancy, thyrotoxicosis)
	Pansystolic	Mitral regurgitation (MR)	Functional MR due to dilatation of mitral valve annulus
			Valvular MR: rheumatic fever, infective endocarditis, mitral valve prolapse, chordal rupture, papillary muscle infarct
		Tricuspid regurgitation (TR)	Functional TR Valvular TR: rheumatic fever, infective endocarditis
		VSD with left to right shunt	Congenital, septal infarct (acquired)
Diastolic	Early diastolic	Aortic regurgitation (AR)	Functional AR: dilatation of valve ring, aortic dissection, cystic medial necrosis (Marfan syndrome)
			Valvular AR: rheumatic fever, infective endocarditis, bicuspid aortic valve
		Pulmonary regurgitation (PR)	Functional PR: dilatation of valve ring, Marfan syndrome, pulmonary hypertension
			Valvular PR: rheumatic fever, carcinoid, Fallot's tetralogy
	Mid-diastolic	Mitral stenosis (MS)	Rheumatic fever, congenital
		Tricuspid stenosis (TS)	Rheumatic fever
		Left and right atrial myxomas	Tumour obstruction of valve orifice in diastole
Continuous		PDA	Congenital
		Arteriovenous fistula	
		Cervical venous hum	

HCM, hypertrophic cardiomyopathy; PDA, patent ductus arteriosus; VSD, ventricular septal defect.

Past medical history

Aim to elicit any history of cardiac disease with particular emphasis on possible causes of a murmur:

- history of rheumatic fever in childhood
- previous cardiac surgery
- myocardial infarction in past – may cause ventricular dilatation and, therefore, functional mitral regurgitation or dysfunction of papillary muscle leading to mitral regurgitation
- family history of cardiac problems or sudden death – as may occur for patients who have HCM
- recent dental procedures or operations – may be a cause of infective endocarditis.

Social history

Ask in particular about:

- smoking – an important risk factor for ischaemic heart disease
- alcohol intake – if excessive may result in dilated cardiomyopathy
- history of intravenous drug abuse.

EXAMINATION OF PATIENTS WHO HAVE A HEART MURMUR

General observation

Look for signs of cardiac failure (i.e. dyspnoea, cyanosis or oedema). Look also for clues indicating the cause of the murmur:

- anaemia – may cause a high-output state or be caused by infective endocarditis
- scars of previous cardiac surgery – median sternotomy, thoracotomy or valvuloplasty scars.

Examine the eyes for retinal haemorrhages (Roth's spots) and conjunctival haemorrhages. These are signs of infective endocarditis.

Fig. 6.2 gives a summary of the findings on examination of a patient who has a heart murmur.

Hands

Look for peripheral stigmas of infective endocarditis:

- Splinter haemorrhages – more than five is pathological
- Osler's nodes (purplish raised papules on finger pulps)
- Janeway lesions (erythematous non-tender lesions on the thenar eminence)
- Finger clubbing.

Cardiovascular system

Pulse

Examine the pulse at both the radial site and the carotid artery. Examples of abnormal pulse due to valvular disease include:

- slow rising or plateau pulse in aortic stenosis
- collapsing or waterhammer pulse in aortic regurgitation or patent ductus arteriosus
- bisferiens pulse in mixed aortic valve disease
- a jerky pulse in HCM.

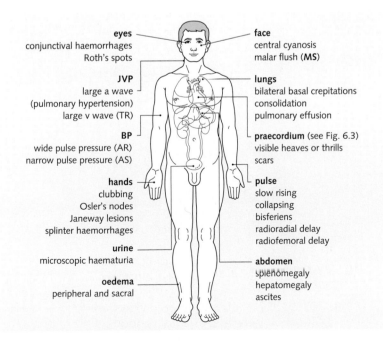

eyes
conjunctival haemorrhages
Roth's spots

face
central cyanosis
malar flush (**MS**)

JVP
large a wave
(pulmonary hypertension)
large v wave (TR)

lungs
bilateral basal crepitations
consolidation
pulmonary effusion

BP
wide pulse pressure (AR)
narrow pulse pressure (AS)

praecordium (see Fig. 6.3)
visible heaves or thrills
scars

hands
clubbing
Osler's nodes
Janeway lesions
splinter haemorrhages

pulse
slow rising
collapsing
bisferiens
radioradial delay
radiofemoral delay

urine
microscopic haematuria

abdomen
splenomegaly
hepatomegaly
ascites

oedema
peripheral and sacral

Fig. 6.2 Possible findings in a patient who has a heart murmur. AS, aortic stenosis; AR, aortic regurgitation; MS, mitral stenosis; TR, tricuspid regurgitation.

Blood pressure

This may also give important clues:

- A narrow pulse pressure associated with hypotension is a sign of severe aortic stenosis.
- A wide pulse pressure may be seen in aortic regurgitation or high-output states.

Jugular venous pressure

Remember the patient must be at 45° with the neck muscles relaxed. The jugular venous pressure is measured as the height of the visible pulsation vertically from the sternal angle. Possible findings include:

- an elevated jugular venous pressure in congestive cardiac failure
- large 'a' waves (see Fig. 23.4) in pulmonary stenosis and pulmonary hypertension
- large 'v' waves – a sign of tricuspid regurgitation.

Praecordium

Remember to look for scars of previous surgery. On palpation, the apex beat is the lowest and most lateral point at which the cardiac impulse can be felt. Possible abnormalities in a patient who has a murmur include:

- displaced apex beat – due to mitral regurgitation and aortic regurgitation
- double apical impulse – due to HCM, also left ventricular aneurysm
- tapping apex beat – due to mitral stenosis
- heaving apex beat – due to aortic stenosis
- thrusting apex beat – due to aortic or mitral regurgitation or any high-output state.

Right-ventricular heave is a sign of right-ventricular strain and may be felt in patients who have right-ventricular failure due to mitral valve disease.

Thrills (or palpable murmurs) may be felt in any of the cardiac areas where the corresponding murmurs are best heard. The positions of valve areas are shown in Fig. 6.3.

Murmurs from valves on the left side of the heart (mitral and aortic) are heard best in expiration. Those from the right side of the heart (pulmonary and tricuspid) are heard best in inspiration.

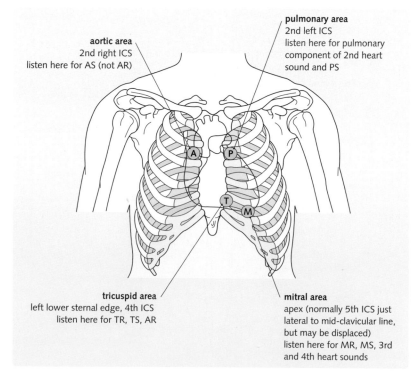

Fig. 6.3 Praecordium, illustrating the position of valve areas. AR, aortic regurgitation; AS, aortic stenosis; ICS, intercostal space; MR, mitral regurgitation; MS, mitral stenosis; PS, pulmonary stenosis; TR, tricuspid regurgitation; TS, tricuspid stenosis.

aortic area
2nd right ICS
listen here for AS (not AR)

pulmonary area
2nd left ICS
listen here for pulmonary component of 2nd heart sound and PS

tricuspid area
left lower sternal edge, 4th ICS
listen here for TR, TS, AR

mitral area
apex (normally 5th ICS just lateral to mid-clavicular line, but may be displaced)
listen here for MR, MS, 3rd and 4th heart sounds

Characteristics of common murmurs are listed in Fig. 6.4.

Cardiac auscultation is difficult – as is the interpretation of heart murmurs. You should listen carefully to the heart sounds of every patient that you examine – and become familiar with the normal cardiac sounds – this will help greatly when you encounter abnormal heart sounds and murmurs.

Peripheral vascular system

All peripheral pulses should be palpated. Radioradial delay and radiofemoral delay may be found with coarctation of the aorta. Also seen in this condition is discrepancy in the blood pressure taken in each arm. It is important to look for these signs as part of the cardiovascular examination.

It is important to know these characteristics for each of the common murmurs:

- Location at which to listen for the murmur
- Position of the patient for each murmur
- Phase of respiration during which each murmur is best heard
- Nature of the murmur and where it radiates.

Fig. 6.4 Important characteristics of common murmurs

valve lesion	murmur	patient position	phase of respiration	radiation	other features
MS	mid-diastolic, low and rumbling, listen with bell of stethoscope, loud S_1, OS	lying on left side	expiration	none	tapping non-displaced apex; often associated with atrial fibrillation; pulmonary hypertension may occur with loud P_2 and TR
MR	pansystolic, listen with diaphragm of stethoscope, soft S_1	on back at 45 degrees	expiration	to axilla	thrusting, displaced apex, may be associated with atrial fibrillation
AS	ejection systolic murmur, listen with diaphragm, may get reversal of S_2 due to prolonged LV emptying	on back at 45 degrees	expiration	to carotid arteries	heaving, non-displaced apex; slow-rising, low-volume pulse
AR	soft, blowing early diastolic murmur, heard in tricuspid area, soft S_2, may hear Austin Flint murmur, listen with diaphragm	sitting forward	expiration	none	thrusting, displaced apex; waterhammer (collapsing) pulse, wide pulse pressure, Duroziez's sign, Quincke's sign, pistol shot femorals, de Musset's sign

The second heart sound (S_2) has two components: A_2 (aortic value closure) and P_2 (pulmonary valve closure). AS. aortic stenosis; AR, aortic regurgitation; LV, left ventricle; MR mitral regurgitation; MS, mitral stenosis; OS, opening snap; S_1, first heart sound; TR, tricuspid regurgitation.

Peripheral oedema

This may be elicited by applying firm pressure for at least 15 s, eliciting 'pitting oedema' can be painful for the patient – so be careful.

Respiratory system

The chest should be carefully examined. Possible findings include:

- bilateral basal fine end-inspiratory crepitations – suggests pulmonary oedema
- evidence of respiratory tract infection – sepsis may cause a high-output state.

Gastrointestinal system

Important findings include:

- hepatomegaly or ascites, seen in right-sided heart failure or congestive cardiac failure
- splenomegaly, a feature of infective endocarditis.

Dipstick test of the urine should always be performed as part of the bedside examination. Microscopic haematuria is a common finding in patients who have infective endocarditis.

INVESTIGATION OF PATIENTS WHO HAVE A HEART MURMUR

An algorithm for the investigation of heart murmur is given in Fig. 6.5.

Blood tests

These include:

- full blood count – anaemia may be seen as a sign of chronic disease in a patient who has infective endocarditis and is also a cause of hyperdynamic state; a leucocytosis is also a feature of infective endocarditis
- urea, creatinine and electrolytes – may be deranged in patients who have cardiac failure as a result of poor renal perfusion or diuretic therapy
- liver function tests – these may be abnormal in patients who have hepatic congestion secondary to cardiac failure
- blood cultures – at least three sets should be taken before commencement of antibiotic therapy in all patients in whom infective endocarditis is suspected
- ESR and C-reactive protein (CRP) – these are markers of inflammation or infection and are useful in monitoring treatment of infective endocarditis.

Chest radiography

This may reveal an abnormal cardiac shadow (e.g. large left atrium and prominent pulmonary vessels in mitral stenosis, enlarged left ventricle in mitral or aortic regurgitation, or the abnormal aortic shadow in coarctation).

Abnormality in the lung fields may also be seen (e.g. pulmonary oedema, pulmonary effusion).

Electrocardiography

The 12-lead ECG may give useful information:

- Atrial fibrillation may be a sign of mitral valve disease.
- Left-ventricular strain pattern may be seen in aortic stenosis.
- P mitrale may be seen in the ECG if there is pulmonary hypertension secondary to valve disease (as occurs in severe mitral stenosis).

Echocardiography

Transthoracic echocardiography

Transthoracic echocardiography enables the valves to be visualized and pressure gradients across them to be assessed. Left-ventricular function and pulmonary artery pressure can be estimated. The presence of ventricular septal defect or patent ductus arteriosus may be more accurately assessed by cardiac catheterization, but they may be visualized using echocardiography.

Transoesophageal echocardiography

Transoesophageal echocardiography is very useful because it gives very detailed information on structures that are difficult to see using transthoracic echocardiography. Examples of its uses include:

- assessment of prosthetic valves
- detailed evaluation of the mitral valve before mitral valve repair.

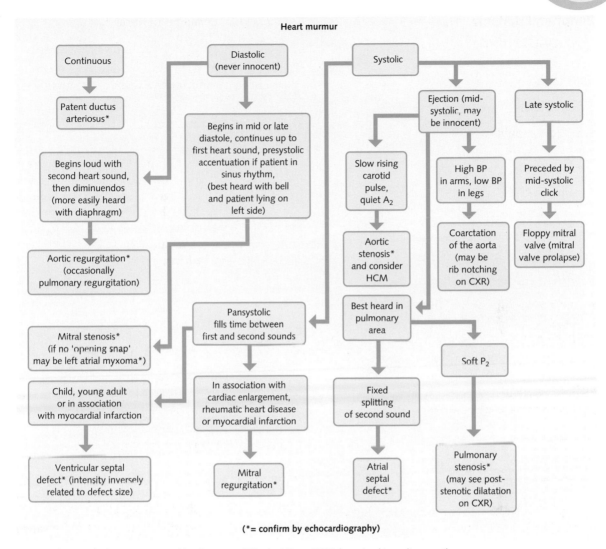

Fig. 6.5 Algorithm for heart murmur. BP, blood pressure; CXR, chest X-ray; HCM, hypertrophic cardiomyopathy.

Cardiac catheterization

Before valve replacement this is performed to obtain information about the:

- presence of coexisting coronary-artery disease

- degree of pulmonary hypertension in patients who have mitral valve disease.

This investigation can also be used to assess the severity of the left-to-right shunt in patients who have ventricular or atrial septal defects.

High blood pressure

A person is hypertensive if three sets of blood pressure measurements taken over at least a 3-month period are higher than 140/90 mmHg.

DIFFERENTIAL DIAGNOSIS

Systemic hypertension may be classified as:

- primary (essential) hypertension, for which there is no identified cause. This accounts for 95% of cases
- secondary hypertension, for which there is a clear cause (Fig. 7.1).

HISTORY TO FOCUS ON THE DIFFERENTIAL DIAGNOSIS OF HIGH BLOOD PRESSURE

Presenting complaint

Hypertensive patients are often asymptomatic. Occasionally they complain of headaches, tinnitus, recurrent epistaxis or dizziness. In this situation a detailed systems review may reveal clues as to a possible cause of hypertension:

- Weight loss or gain, tremor, hair loss, heat intolerance or feeling cold may suggest the presence of thyroid disease.
- Paroxysmal palpitations, sweating, headaches or collapse may indicate the possibility of a phaeochromocytoma.

Ask the patient about symptoms that may indicate the presence of complications of hypertension such as:

- dyspnoea, orthopnoea or ankle oedema suggesting cardiac failure
- chest pain indicating ischaemic heart disease
- unilateral weakness or visual disturbance (either persistent or transient) suggesting cerebrovascular disease.

Past medical history

To gain information about a condition that has so many varied causes it is crucial to ask about all previous illnesses and operations. Examples include:

- recurrent urinary tract infections, especially in childhood, may lead to chronic pyelonephritis, a common cause of renal failure
- a history of asthma may reveal chronic corticosteroid intake, leading to Cushing's syndrome
- thyroid surgery in the past
- evidence of peripheral vascular disease (e.g. leg claudication or previous vascular surgery may suggest the possibility of underlying renovascular disease).

Drug history

A careful history of all drugs being taken regularly is needed, including the use of proprietary analgesics (e.g. aspirin, non-steroidal anti-inflammatory drugs – a possible cause of renal disease).

Family history

Essential hypertension is a multifactorial disease requiring both genetic and environmental inputs.

Fig. 7.1 Causes of secondary hypertension

Mechanism	Pathology
Renal	Renal parenchymal disease (e.g. chronic atrophic pyelonephritis, chronic glomerulonephritis), renal artery stenosis, renin-producing tumours, primary sodium retention
Endocrine	Acromegaly, hypo- and hyperthyroidism, hypercalcaemia, adrenal cortex disorders (e.g. Cushing's disease, Conn's syndrome, congenital adrenal hyperplasia), adrenal medulla disorders (e.g. phaeochromocytoma)
Vascular disease	Coarctation of the aorta
Other	Hypertension of pregnancy, carcinoid syndrome
Increased intravascular volume	Polycythaemia (primary or secondary)
Drugs	Alcohol, oral contraceptives, monoamine oxidase inhibitors, glucocorticoids
Psychogenic	Stress

A family history of hypertension is, therefore, not an uncommon finding in these patients. Some secondary causes of hypertension have a genetic component:

- Adult polycystic kidney disease is an autosomal dominant condition associated with hypertension, renal failure and cerebral artery aneurysms.
- Phaeochromocytoma may occur as part of a multiple endocrine neoplasia syndrome (MEN 2, autosomal dominant) associated with medullary carcinoma of the thyroid and hyperparathyroidism.

Social history

Smoking, like hypertension, is a risk factor for ischaemic heart disease. Excessive alcohol intake can cause hypertension.

EXAMINATION OF PATIENTS WHO HAVE HIGH BLOOD PRESSURE

When performing the examination, look for:

- signs of end-organ damage (i.e. cardiac failure, ischaemic heart disease, peripheral artery disease, cerebrovascular disease and renal impairment)
- signs of an underlying cause of hypertension.

Blood pressure

Important points to note are that:

- the patient should be seated comfortably – preferably for 5 min before measurement of blood pressure in a quiet warm setting
- the correct cuff size should be used – if it is too small a spuriously high reading will result
- the manometer should be correctly calibrated
- the bladder should be inflated to 20 mmHg above systolic blood pressure
- systolic blood pressure is recorded as the point during bladder deflation where regular sounds can be heard. Systolic blood pressure can also be measured as the pressure at which the palpated distal pulse disappears
- diastolic blood pressure is recorded as the point at which the sounds disappear (Korotkoff phase V). In children and pregnant women muffling of the sounds is used as the diastolic blood pressure (Korotkoff phase IV).

When performing the initial blood pressure measurements, measure blood pressure in both arms. A marked difference suggests coarctation of the aorta.

The blood pressure in some patients goes up when they see a doctor – this is 'white coat hypertension'.

Ambulatory blood pressure monitoring can help in the diagnosis of spurious 'white coat hypertension', and also establish efficacy of blood pressure control in patients on treatment

Cardiovascular examination

Examine the pulses, considering the following:

- Rate – tachycardia or bradycardia may indicate underlying thyroid disease
- Rhythm – atrial fibrillation may occur as a result of hypertensive heart disease
- Symmetry – compare the pulses; radioradial delay is a sign of coarctation as is the finding of abnormally weak foot pulses.

Bear in mind that:

- weak or absent peripheral pulses along with cold extremities suggest peripheral vascular disease
- jugular venous pressure may be elevated in congestive cardiac failure; a complication of hypertension
- a displaced apex is seen in left-ventricular failure due to dilatation of the left ventricle
- mitral regurgitation may occur secondary to dilatation of the valve ring that occurs during left-ventricular dilatation
- in patients who have aortic coarctation, bruits may be heard over the scapulas and a systolic murmur may be heard below the left clavicle.

Respiratory system

Bilateral basal crepitations of pulmonary oedema may be heard on examination of the respiratory system.

Gastrointestinal system

Hepatomegaly and ascites may be seen in patients with congestive cardiac failure. Abdominal aortic aneurysm must be looked for because it is a manifestation of generalized atherosclerosis. Palpable kidneys may be evident in individuals who have polycystic kidney disease. A renal artery bruit may be heard in patients with renal artery stenosis.

Limbs

Peripheral oedema is a sign of congestive cardiac failure or underlying renal disease.

Eyes

Hypertensive retinopathy

A detailed examination of the fundi is crucial in all patients who have hypertension because it provides valuable information about the severity of the hypertension (Fig. 7.2). Patients exhibiting grade III or IV hypertensive retinopathy have accelerated or malignant hypertension and need urgent treatment.

Fig. 7.3 highlights the features of the different grades of hypertensive retinopathy.

Other findings on examination

When examining a patient who has a disorder that has many possible causes, a thorough examination of all systems is vital. Remember to look out for signs of thyroid disease, Cushing's disease, acromegaly, renal impairment, etc.

INVESTIGATION OF PATIENTS WHO HAVE HIGH BLOOD PRESSURE

Algorithms for the investigation of high blood pressure are given in Fig. 7.4. Look for evidence of end-organ damage and possible underlying causes.

As the treatment of hypertension is lifelong therapy with one or more drugs, it is important that the diagnosis is made correctly. Three elevated blood-pressure measurements (>140/90 mmHg) over a 3-month period confirm the diagnosis; however, a single very elevated reading is also acceptable to establish the diagnosis and initiate treatment.

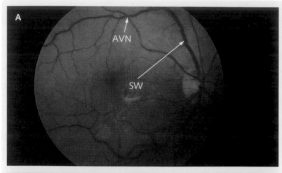

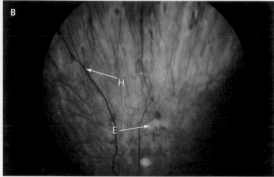

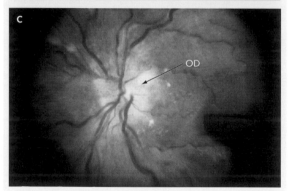

Fig. 7.2 Stages of hypertensive retinopathy. (A) Grade II, showing silver wiring (SW) and arteriovenous nipping (AVN) where an artery crossing above a vein causes apparent compression of the underlying vein. (B) Grade III, showing evidence of haemorrhages (H) and exudates (E). (C) Papilloedema – the optic disc (OD) is swollen and oedematous – a sign of malignant hypertension.

Fig. 7.3 Features of hypertensive retinopathy on ophthalmoscopy

Grade	Features
I	Narrowing of the arteriolar lumen occurs giving the classical 'silver wiring' effect
II	Sclerosis of the adventitia and thickening of the muscular wall of the arteries leads to compression of underlying veins and 'arteriovenous nipping'
III	Rupture of small vessels leading to haemorrhages and exudates
IV	Papilloedema (plus signs of grades I–IV) OD

- Full blood count – polycythaemia may be present. Macrocytosis may be seen in hypothyroidism; anaemia may be a result of chronic renal failure
- Blood glucose – elevated blood glucose may be seen in diabetes mellitus or in Cushing's disease
- Thyroid function
- Blood lipid profile – like hypertension, an important risk factor for ischaemic heart disease.

If treatment of hypertension with angiotensin-converting enzyme inhibitors causes a rise in serum creatinine, consider renal artery stenosis.

Urinalysis

Look for protein casts or red blood cells – a sign of underlying renal disease.

Electrocardiography

There may be evidence of left-ventricular hypertrophy. Features of left-ventricular hypertrophy, shown in Fig. 7.5, are:

- tall R waves in lead V6 (>25 mm)
- R wave in V5 plus S wave in V2 >35 mm
- deep S wave in lead V2
- inverted T waves in lateral leads (i.e. I, AVL, V5 and V6).

Blood tests

The following blood tests may help in the diagnosis:

- Electrolytes and renal function – many patients who have hypertension may be treated with diuretics and, therefore, may have hypokalaemia or hyponatraemia as a result. Renal impairment as a result of hypertension or its treatment must be excluded

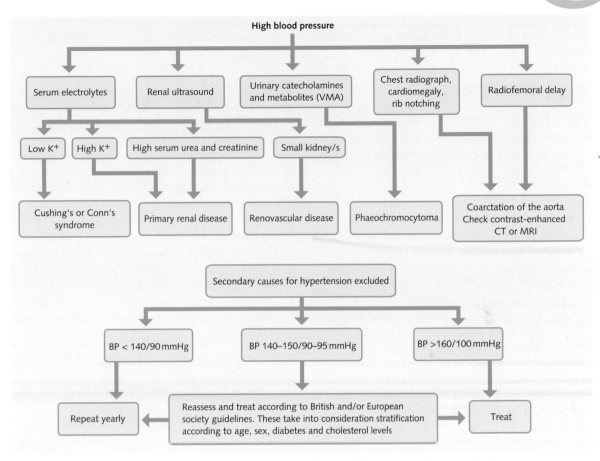

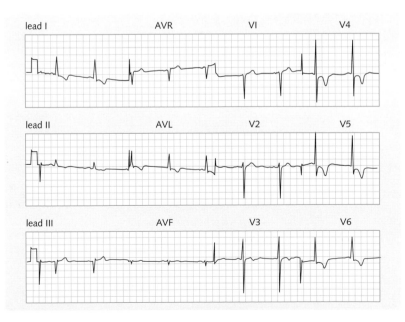

Fig. 7.4 Algorithm for high blood pressure. BP, blood pressure; CT, computed tomography; MRI, magnetic resonance imaging; VMA, vanillylmandelic acid.

Fig. 7.5 Electrocardiographic features of left-ventricular hypertrophy (LVH). Note the three cardinal features indicating LVH: R wave in V5 plus S wave in V2 exceeds seven large squares; the R wave in V6 and S wave in V2 are greater than five large squares; T wave inversion in lateral leads V4–V6.

There may be evidence of an old myocardial infarction or of rhythm disturbance especially atrial fibrillation.

Chest radiography

Look for:

- an enlarged left ventricle – seen on the chest radiograph as an enlarged cardiac shadow. The normal ratio of cardiac width to thoracic width is 1:2
- evidence of coarctation of the aorta – this is seen as poststenotic dilatation of the aorta with an indentation above producing the reversed figure three, along with rib notching due to dilatation of the posterior intercostal arteries.

Echocardiography

This investigation is used to:

- reveal left-ventricular hypertrophy
- reveal poor left-ventricular function

- show any ventricular-wall-motion abnormalities suggestive of old myocardial infarction (MI).

INVESTIGATIONS TO EXCLUDE SECONDARY HYPERTENSION

The above investigations may point to possible underlying causes of secondary hypertension, but they are not exhaustive. It would not, however, be cost-effective to investigate all hypertensive patients for these disorders, because over 95% of cases of hypertension are primary.

Careful selection of patients who are more likely to have secondary hypertension is, therefore, needed before embarking on more detailed and invasive investigations. Secondary hypertension is more likely in patients who are under 35 years of age and also in patients who have:

- symptoms of malignant hypertension (i.e. severe headaches, nausea and vomiting, blood pressure >180/100 mmHg or papilloedema)

Fig. 7.6 Investigation of secondary hypertension

Underlying cause	Investigation	Notes/Result
Renal parenchymal disease	24-hour creatinine clearance 24-hour protein excretion Renal ultrasound Renal biopsy	↓ ↑ Bilateral small kidneys In some cases
Renal artery stenosis	Renal ultrasound Radionucleotide studies using DTPA Renal angiography or MRI angiography	Often asymmetrical kidneys Decreased uptake on affected side; this effect is highlighted by administration of an ACE inhibitor
Phaeochromocytoma	24-hour urine catecholamines CT scan of abdomen MIBG scan	↑, VMA measurements now rarely used Tumour is often large To identify extra-adrenal tumours (seen in 10% cases)
Cushing's disease	24-hour urinary free cortisol Dexamethasone suppression test 09:00 and 24:00 blood cortisol Adrenal CT scan Pituitary MRI scan Chest X-ray	↑ Low-dose 48-hour test initially, high-dose test to rule out ectopic source of ACTH Reveals loss of circadian rhythm in Cushing's disease May show adrenal tumaur May show enlarged pituitary May show oat cell carcinoma of bronchus (ectopic ACTH)

ACE, angiotensin-converting enzyme; ACTH, adrenocorticotrophic hormone; CT, computed tomography; DTPA, diethylenetriamine penta-acetate; MIBG, meta-iodobenzylguanidine; MRI, magnetic resonance imaging; VMA, vanillylmandelic acid.

- evidence of end-organ damage (i.e. grade III or IV retinopathy, raised serum creatinine or cardiac failure)
- signs of secondary causes (e.g. hypokalaemia in the absence of diuretics, signs of coarctation, abdominal bruit, symptoms of phaeochromocytoma, family history of renal disease or stroke at a young age)
- poorly controlled blood pressure despite medical therapy.

Investigations for secondary hypertension are listed in Fig. 7.6.

Failure of hypertension to respond to treatment might be because there is an underlying secondary cause or because of lack of compliance with therapy.

Fever associated with a cardiac symptom or sign

Objectives

By the end of this chapter you should:

- be able to take a history and examine a patient that presents with fever, with specific relevance to symptoms and signs of cardiovascular disease
- understand the differential diagnosis of fever associated with cardiovascular disease
- understand the appropriate investigations to be used in the management of a patient with fever and cardiovascular symptoms.

DIFFERENTIAL DIAGNOSIS

Some very serious and potentially fatal cardiac conditions are accompanied by fever. It is, therefore, important to have at hand a working list of differential diagnoses when presented with such a case.

The differential diagnosis includes:

- infective endocarditis – bacterial or fungal infection within the heart (Fig. 8.1)
- myocarditis – involvement of the myocardium in an inflammatory process, which is usually infectious
- pericarditis – inflammation of the pericardium, which may be infective, postmyocardial infarction or autoimmune
- other rare conditions, such as cardiac myxoma.

The fever may be of non-cardiac origin.

Rare conditions

Cardiac myxomas:

- are benign primary tumours of the heart
- are most often located in the atria
- may present with a wide variety of symptoms (e.g. dyspnoea, fever, weight loss and syncope)
- can cause complications, such as thromboembolic phenomena or sudden death

- are diagnosed by echocardiography
- are treated with anticoagulation to prevent thromboembolic phenomena and resection (they may recur if incompletely resected).

In the viva, a well-presented list of differential diagnoses implies that you can think laterally and adapt your knowledge of cardiac conditions to fit a clinical scenario.

Whenever presenting a list of differential diagnoses, start with either the most dangerous or the most common disorder. Leave the rare conditions to the end (even though these are invariably the ones that immediately spring to mind).

HISTORY TO FOCUS ON THE DIFFERENTIAL DIAGNOSIS OF FEVER

When presented with a set of symptoms that cover a potentially huge set of differential diagnoses, it is important to be systematic. Remember that sepsis is a common cause of atrial fibrillation and flutter. Patients who have sepsis may, therefore, present with fever and palpitations.

Fig. 8.1 Duke criteria for the diagnosis of infective endocarditis (IE)

Criteria	Description
Major	
A	Positive blood culture for IE

	1 – Typical microorganism consistent with IE from 2 separate blood cultures, as noted below:
	   • viridans streptococci, *Streptococcus bovis*, or HACEK*
	     group, or
	   • community-acquired *Staphylococcus aureus* or enterococci,
	     in the absence of a primary focus
	or

	2 – Microorganisms consistent with IE from persistently positive blood cultures defined as:
	   • two positive cultures of blood samples drawn >12 h
	     apart, or
	   • all of three or a majority of four separate cultures of blood
	     (with first and last sample drawn 1 h apart)

B	Evidence of endocardial involvement
	1 – Positive echocardiogram for IE defined as: oscillating intracardiac mass on valve or supporting structures, in the path of regurgitant jets, or on implanted material in the absence of an alternative anatomic explanation, or abscess, or new partial dehiscence of prosthetic valve or
	2 – New valvular regurgitation (worsening or changing of preexisting murmur not sufficient)
Minor	• Predisposition: predisposing heart condition or intravenous drug use • Fever: temperature > 38.0°C (100.4°F) • Vascular phenomena: major arterial emboli, septic pulmonary infarcts, mycotic aneurysm, intracranial haemorrhage, conjunctival haemorrhages, and Janeway lesions • Immunologic phenomena: glomerulonephritis, Osler's nodes, Roth spots, and rheumatoid factor • Microbiological evidence: positive blood culture but does not meet a major criterion as noted above or serological evidence of active infection with organism consistent with IE • Echocardiographic findings: consistent with IE but do not meet a major criterion as noted above

Clinical criteria for infective endocarditis requires:
- Two major criteria, or
- One major and three minor criteria, or
- Five minor criteria

*HACEK group: *Haemophilus* sp, *Actinobacillus actinomycetemcomitans*, *Cardiobacterium hominis*, *Eikenella corrodens*, *Kingella kingae*

Presenting complaint

Common presenting complaints include:

- fever – ask when it started and whether the patient can think of any precipitating factors (e.g. an operation or dental work)

- chest pain – to differentiate between ischaemic and pericarditic pain, for example, establish the exact nature of the pain, where it radiates, duration and exacerbating factors (Fig. 8.2)
- palpitations – ask about rate and rhythm to obtain information about the likely nature of

Fig. 8.2 Important features of ischaemic and pericarditic pain

Condition	Pericarditis	Ischaemia
Location	Praecordium	Retrosternal ± radiation to left arm, throat or jaw
Quality	Sharp, pleuritic (may be dull)	Pressure pain (usually builds up)
Duration	Hours to days	Minutes, usually resolving (occasionally lasts hours)
Relationship to exercise	No	Yes, unless unstable angina or myocardial infarction
Relationship to posture	Worse when recumbent, relieved when sitting forward	Usually no effect

the palpitations. Also ask about the possible complications of palpitations (e.g. dyspnoea, angina, dizziness).

Past medical history

It is crucial to obtain a detailed past medical history. In particular the following aspects of the past medical history are important in these patients:

- Recent dental work – this is a common source of bacteraemia and cause of infective endocarditis.
- Recent operations – these may also cause transient bacteraemia (e.g. gastrointestinal surgery, genitourinary surgery or even endoscopic investigations).
- History of rheumatic fever – although rare in the developed world now, this condition was common in the early twentieth century and is the cause of valve damage in many elderly patients. Such abnormal valves are vulnerable to colonization by bacteria.
- Previous myocardial infarction – a possible cause of pericarditis and Dressler's syndrome (a non-specific, possibly autoimmune, inflammatory response to cardiac necrosis in surgery).
- Recent viral infection (e.g. a sore throat or a cold) – myocarditis and pericarditis are commonly caused by viral infection.

Drug history

Ask about any recent antibiotics taken – obtain exact details of drugs and doses. Remember that some drugs may cause pericarditis, for example penicillin (associated with hypereosinophilia), hydralazine, procainamide and isoniazid.

Social history

Ask about:

- history of intravenous drug abuse, which is a risk factor for infective endocarditis
- risk factors for human immunodeficiency virus infection, which may be associated with infection due to unusual organisms
- smoking, which is a common cause for recurrent chest infection or myocardial infarction.

EXAMINATION OF PATIENTS WHO HAVE A FEVER ASSOCIATED WITH A CARDIAC SYMPTOM OR SIGN

Fig. 8.2 highlights the important features on examination of a patient who has fever and a cardiac sign or symptom.

Temperature

Examine the temperature chart to establish not only the severity of the fever, but also its trends (i.e. increasing, decreasing, cyclical variation, etc.).

Hands

Look for signs of infective endocarditis:

- Clubbing
- Osler's nodes (tender purplish nodules on the finger pulps)
- Janeway lesions (erythematous areas on palms)
- Splinter haemorrhages – up to four can be considered to be normal. The most common

cause for a lesion that has the same appearance as a splinter haemorrhage is trauma, so they are common in keen gardeners.

All these are signs of vasculitis and may be found in other conditions causing vasculitis (e.g. autoimmune disease).

Facies

Look for:

- conjunctival haemorrhages and Roth's spots (retinal haemorrhages) – both signs of infective endocarditis
- central cyanosis – this may be a sign of a chest infection or cardiac failure
- a vasculitic rash (e.g. the butterfly rash of systemic lupus erythematosus).

Cardiovascular system

Pulse

Check the:

- rate and rhythm – may reveal underlying tachyarrhythmia (e.g. atrial fibrillation or, more commonly, sinus tachycardia – a common finding in a patient who has pyrexia)
- quality of pulse – may reveal an underlying valve abnormality (e.g. waterhammer or collapsing pulse suggesting aortic regurgitation caused by endocarditis affecting the aortic valve).

Blood pressure

Hypotension may be found suggesting septic shock or cardiac failure.

A large pericardial effusion causing tamponade may result in pulsus paradoxus, which is an exaggeration of the normal variation of the blood pressure during respiration (i.e. the blood pressure falls during inspiration; a fall greater than 10 mmHg is abnormal).

Jugular venous pressure

Look for:

- Kussmaul's sign – jugular venous pressure (JVP) increases with inspiration (normally, it falls), as seen in cases where pericardial effusion leads to cardiac tamponade

- Friedreich's sign – a rapid collapse of the JVP during diastole seen in aortic regurgitation. The JVP may be elevated due to cardiac failure.

Praecordium

Look for scars of previous valve replacement (prosthetic valves are more prone to infective endocarditis). The scar for these operations is the median sternotomy scar. Do not forget the mitral valvotomy scar under the left breast. Closed mitral valvotomy has been superseded by mitral valvuloplasty, which is undertaken via the femoral artery. However, there are still patients who have had closed mitral valvotomy to treat mitral stenosis in the past and these are also vulnerable to infective endocarditis.

Listen for:

- murmurs, especially those of valvular incompetence caused by infective endocarditis
- prosthetic valve sounds
- pericardial rub – this may be heard in patients who have pericarditis and has been described as the squeak of new leather. It is best heard with the diaphragm of the stethoscope and can be distinguished from a heart murmur because its timing with the heart cycle often varies from beat to beat and may appear and disappear from one day to the next.

Respiratory system

Examine carefully for signs of infection such as bronchial breathing, a pleural rub or pleural effusion.

Gastrointestinal system

Possible findings include:

- splenomegaly, which is an important finding because it is a sign of infective endocarditis
- hepatomegaly, which may be found as a consequence of cardiac failure or of viral infection (e.g. infectious mononucleosis).

Skin

Infective endocarditis and many viral infections may be associated with a petechial rash.

An algorithm for the investigation of fever is given in Fig. 8.3.

Blood tests

Blood cultures

This is the most important diagnostic test in infective endocarditis.

At least three sets of blood cultures should be taken, if possible 1 h apart, from different sites before commencing antibiotics. This enables isolation of the causative organism in over 98% of cases of bacterial endocarditis. Therapy is often started immediately after this and can then be modified when the blood culture results are available.

Full blood count

A full blood count may reveal:

- anaemia of chronic disease, which is commonly seen in patients who have infective endocarditis
- a leucocytosis, which is an indicator of infection or inflammation
- thrombocytopenia, which may accompany disseminated intravascular coagulopathy in cases of severe sepsis.

Other blood tests

These include:

- antistreptolysin O titres – may be useful in cases of rheumatic fever
- monospot test if Epstein-Barr virus infection is suspected as a possible cause of viral myocarditis

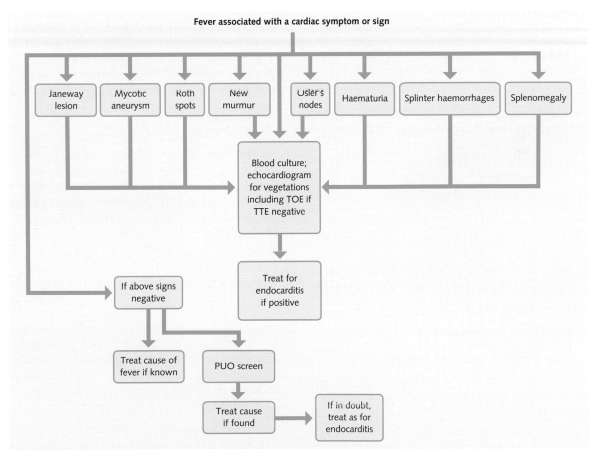

Fig. 8.3 Algorithm for fever. PUO, pyrexia of unknown origin; TOE, transoesophageal echocardiography; TTE, transthoracic echocardiography.

- clotting screen – clotting may be deranged in cases of sepsis associated with disseminated intravascular coagulation (DIC)
- renal function tests – may be abnormal in infective endocarditis because the associated vasculitis may involve the kidneys causing glomerulonephritis. Autoimmune disease may also cause renal dysfunction and is a cause of pericarditis and myocarditis
- liver function tests – abnormal in many viral infections
- erythrocyte sedimentation rate and C-reactive protein measurements – these inflammatory markers are a sensitive indicator of the presence of infection or inflammation. They are also invaluable as markers of the response to treatment. Because C-reactive protein has a short half-life (approximately 8 h) it is often a more sensitive marker of disease activity than the erythrocyte sedimentation rate
- viral titres – taken in the acute and convalescent phase of the illness and may reveal the cause of pericarditis or myocarditis. If viral illness is suspected, throat swabs and faecal culture are also appropriate investigations to isolate the organism.

Urinalysis

No examination of a cardiovascular patient is complete without dipstick testing of the urine to look for microscopic haematuria. This is an extremely sensitive test for infective endocarditis and must not be forgotten. Urine microscopy almost always reveals red blood cells in infective endocarditis. Proteinuria may also be found.

Electrocardiography

In patients who have pericarditis the ECG may show characteristic ST segment elevation. This differs from that seen in myocardial infarction because it is:

- concave
- present in all leads
- associated with upright T waves.

Eventually, with time, the ST segments may flatten or invert but, unlike infarction, there is no loss of R wave height.

Myocarditis may be associated with atrial arrhythmias or interventricular conduction defects. Rarely complete heart block may occur.

Chest radiography

This may reveal an underlying cause of cardiac disease:

- Pneumonia – a possible cause of atrial fibrillation
- Lung tumour – may invade the pericardium causing pericardial effusion
- Cardiac failure – an enlarged cardiac shadow and pulmonary oedema may be seen in patients who have valve disease or myocarditis
- A globular heart shadow – characteristic of a pericardial effusion
- Calcified heart valves – may be visible in a patient who has a history of rheumatic fever.

Transthoracic echocardiography

Transthoracic echocardiography is a very useful investigation in the patient who has fever and a cardiac symptom or sign:

- Left-ventricular function can be accurately assessed – in myocarditis this is found to be globally reduced (in patients who have left-ventricular failure due to ischaemic heart disease the left ventricle often shows regional dysfunction according to the site of the vascular lesion)
- Valve lesions may be identified and in cases of infective endocarditis the vegetations may be visualized on the valve leaflets. It is important to remember, however, that infective endocarditis cannot be excluded by the absence of vegetations on echocardiography. This investigation is by no means 100% sensitive and blood cultures remain the most important investigation for this condition.

Transoesophageal echocardiography

Transoesophageal echocardiography is more sensitive than transthoracic echocardiography because the resolution is much better. It allows a more detailed examination to be made and is especially useful in cases where transthoracic echocardiography does not provide adequate imaging, for example:

- prosthetic heart valves – the acoustic shadows cast by these make imaging with transthoracic echocardiography very difficult

- localization of vegetations – transoesophageal echocardiography will visualize vegetations in many cases of infective endocarditis.

Pericardiocentesis

This may be appropriate if a pericardial effusion is found at echocardiography. The procedure is performed by an experienced operator and uses echocardiography as a guide for positioning of a catheter in the pericardial space. An ECG lead is often attached to the needle when attempting to enter the pericardium and will show an injury current (with ST elevation) if the myocardium is touched so enabling myocardial puncture to be avoided. Pericardiocentesis may be:

- therapeutic – if it relieves cardiac tamponade
- diagnostic – if the pericardial fluid can be cultured to reveal an infective organism.

DISEASES AND DISORDERS

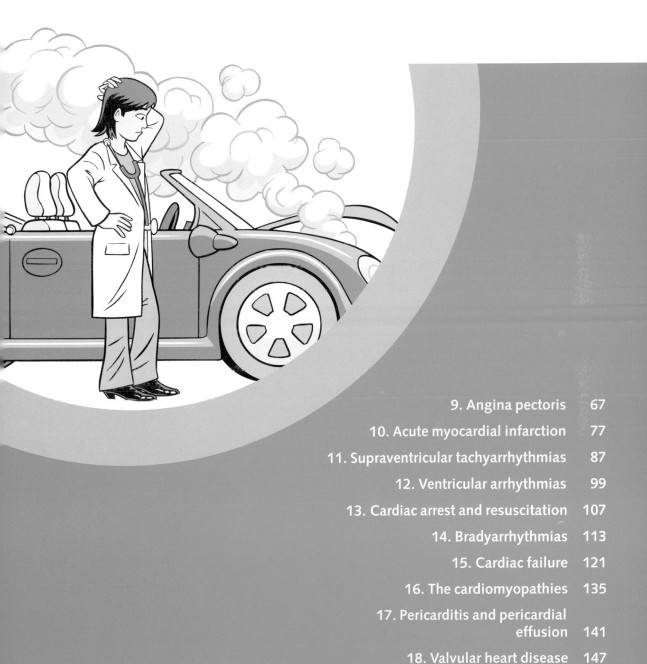

Angina pectoris

9

Objectives

By the end of this chapter you should:

- understand the major modifiable risk factors for coronary artery disease
- understand the difference between stable and unstable angina
- be able to identify the ECG changes that occur during stable and unstable angina
- be able to list the main drug groups used in the treatment of angina
- understand the antiplatelet agents that are used during and after percutaneous intervention
- understand the advantages and disadvantages of both percutaneous intervention (PCI) and coronary artery bypass graft (CABG) for coronary revascularization.

DEFINITION OF ANGINA PECTORIS

Angina pectoris is a severe crushing pain felt in the anterior chest, commonly radiating to the left arm and jaw. The pain is caused by coronary arterial insufficiency leading to intermittent myocardial ischaemia. (Ischaemia refers to the effect of reduced delivery of oxygen and nutrients to an organ or cell.)

PATHOPHYSIOLOGY OF ANGINA PECTORIS

Myocardial ischaemia occurs when oxygen demand exceeds supply (Fig. 9.1).

Supply may be reduced for a number of reasons:

- Stenotic atheromatous disease of epicardial coronary arteries – the most common cause of angina
- Thrombosis within the arteries
- Spasm of normal coronary arteries
- Inflammation – arteritis.

Demand may be increased for a number of reasons:

- In conditions requiring increased cardiac output – exercise, stress or thyrotoxicosis
- In conditions necessitating greater cardiac work to maintain an adequate output – aortic stenosis

- In conditions where peripheral vascular resistance is increased – hypertension.

The rest of this chapter discusses angina due to atherosclerotic narrowing of the coronary arteries because this is the most common cause of angina.

RISK FACTORS FOR CORONARY ARTERY DISEASE

Any modifiable risk factors should be sought and treated to reduce the risk of disease progression and eventual myocardial infarction (Fig. 9.2).

CLINICAL FEATURES OF ANGINA PECTORIS

Symptoms

These include:

- chest pain – classically a tight, crushing, bandlike pain across the centre of the chest. The pain may radiate to the left arm, throat or jaw. Precipitating factors include exercise, anxiety and cold air. As the coronary artery narrowing worsens, the amount of exertion required to produce angina reduces and the pain may occur even at rest or on minimal exertion. Relieving factors include rest and nitrates

Fig. 9.1 Factors involved in the development of ischaemia

Supply factor	Comments
Coronary blood flow	Decreased by fixed stenosis (e.g. atheroma, thrombus); vascular tone – depends on a number of factors including endothelium-dependent relaxing factor (nitric oxide), prostaglandins and input from the autonomic nervous system
Oxygen-carrying capacity	Reduced in anaemia and carboxyhaemoglobinaemia
Demand factor	**Comments**
Heart rate	Increased by exercise, emotion, tachyarrhythmias, outflow obstruction, hypertension, etc.
Contractility	Decreased by rest and negatively inotropic and chronotropic agents (e.g. β-blockers); increased by exertion and positive inotropes (e.g. adrenaline; epinephrine)
Wall tension	Increased by left ventricular dilatation (e.g. nocturnal angina)

Fig. 9.2 Risk factors for coronary artery disease

Non-modifiable risk factors for coronary artery disease
Age: risk increases with age; older patients have a higher risk and therefore a potentially greater risk reduction if modifiable risk factors are treated
Sex: men > women (incidence in women increases rapidly after menopause)
Family history: this is a strong risk factor even when known genetic diseases (e.g. familial hypercholesterolaemia) are excluded

Modifiable risk factors for coronary artery disease
Hypertension
Diabetes mellitus
Smoking
Hypercholesterolaemia: important studies include CARE (*N Engl J Med* 335), Helsinki Heart Study (*N Engl J Med* 317), LIPID (*N Engl J Med* 339), MRFIT (*JAMA* 248), SSSS (*Lancet* 344) and WOSCOPS (*N Engl J Med* 333)

Other risk factors currently being researched
Fibrinogen
Homocysteine
Low levels of antioxidants
Insulin resistance short of overt diabetes mellitus
Metabolic syndrome

CARE, Cholesterol and Recurrent Events Trial; LIPID, Long-tem Intervention with Pravastatin in Ischaemic Heart Disease; MRFIT, Multiple Risk Factor Intervention Trial; SSSS, Scandinavian Simvastatin Survival Study; WOSCOPS, West of Scotland Coronary Prevention Study.

- dyspnoea – often experienced. This occurs when the ischaemic myocardium becomes dysfunctional with an increase in left-ventricular filling pressure and, if severe, progression to pulmonary oedema
- fatigue – may be a manifestation of angina, which should be suspected if it occurs abnormally early into exercise and resolves rapidly at rest or to nitrates.

Most patients will have no obvious signs on examination. The patient may be breathless or sweaty and tachycardia all due to overactivity of the sympathetic nervous system. There also might be evidence of an underlying cause:

- Hypertension
- Corneal arcus or xanthelasma – suggesting hypercholesterolaemia.

Important points when diagnosing angina are:

- a sudden increase in exertional angina may be due to rupture of an atheromatous plaque in the coronary artery, which causes a steep decrease in its luminal diameter, and may even cause intermittent occlusion of the vessel. This condition may progress to myocardial infarction
- oesophageal pain is also relieved by nitrates
- chest pain on exertion can also be musculoskeletal in origin – obtain objective evidence of myocardial ischaemia before giving an opinion
- any form of chest discomfort, even if atypical, could be angina, especially if it is related to effort
- nicotine staining of the fingers in heavy smokers
- aortic stenosis
- abnormal tachyarrhythmia
- anaemia.

There may be evidence of cardiac failure (third heart sound, raised jugular venous pressure, bilateral basal crepitations and possibly peripheral oedema due to fluid retention).

INVESTIGATION OF ANGINA PECTORIS

Resting electrocardiography

Resting ECG may be normal even in individuals who have very severe angina. Signs of angina on the resting ECG include:

- T wave flattening
- T wave inversion
- ST segment depression
- partial or complete left bundle branch block.

Stress testing

There are many methods of stress testing. All aim to place the myocardium under stress and increase oxygen demand and, therefore, precipitate ischaemia, which can be detected in a number of ways.

Remember that precipitation of ischaemia is potentially hazardous and, therefore, all these tests should be performed with facilities for resuscitation close at hand.

Exercise electrocardiography

The patient is made to walk on a treadmill that becomes incrementally faster and steeper at fixed time intervals (the Bruce Protocol). ECG monitoring is used throughout the test and the presence of horizontal ST depression of >1 mm suggests the presence of angina (an ST depression of 2 mm is strongly suggestive of angina). Exercise ECGs are only 70% specific and 70% sensitive and are less reliable in women than men.

Myocardial perfusion imaging – exercise stress

The exercise test is performed as above, but a radionucleotide is injected at peak exercise and the patient is encouraged to continue exercising for at least another 30 s. This allows perfused myocardium to pick up the radionucleotide (any ischaemic myocardium will not pick it up due to poor perfusion). Images of tracer uptake are performed at this stage and also after rest some time later (when the ischaemia has resolved and the affected myocardium has had a chance to take up the tracer). Comparison of the two images provides information on the site of reversible ischaemia. In patients who are unable to exercise adequately due to, for example, peripheral vascular disease, arthritis, chronic obstructive airways disease or asthma, pharmacological agents can be used to simulate vigourous exercise. The drugs used for this include dobutamine and adenosine.

Stress echocardiography

Imaging of the cardiac muscle at rest and immediately after exercise or dobutamine allows accurate definition of areas of irreversible ischaemia (scar or infarct), and reversible ischaemia. In addition, stress echocardiography can give accurate information regarding left-ventricular function and regional-wall-motion abnormalities.

Multi slice CT

Multi slice spiral computed tomography (MSCT) coronary angiography is a relatively new non-invasive technique that can visualize both the lumen and the wall of the coronary arteries. The latest MSCT scanners allow reliable detection of significant obstructive lesions in native coronary arteries in selected patients. Despite significant challenges (calcification in the vessels and irregular heart rhythms being just two), it remains likely that MSCT will become a standard part of the assessment of patients with suspected or known coronary artery disease in the near future.

Coronary angiography

This is the most specific and sensitive test of coronary artery anatomical lesions and, as such, is the 'Gold Standard' in terms of diagnosis. Coronary angiography is used in patients who have positive stress tests and in patients who have negative stress tests in whom the diagnosis of angina is still suspected as stress tests may give false-negative results.

An arterial puncture is made under local anaesthetic in the femoral or radial artery and a guide-wire is passed under X-ray control to the aortic root. A series of pre-shaped catheters is used to locate the right and left coronary ostia and radio-opaque dye is injected into each in turn. Images are taken from several angles to obtain a full view of all branches of the two coronary arteries.

Information on left-ventricular function is obtained by measurement of the left-ventricular end-diastolic pressure (this is elevated in patients with poor left-ventricular function). Injection of dye into the left-ventricle allows the pattern of left-ventricular contraction can be seen and gives an assessment of function.

It is important to remember that coronary angiography is invasive and there is a small risk of morbidity and mortality associated with the procedure.

Syndrome X

This is the term given to a group of patients (mostly middle-aged women) with the following characteristics:

- Symptoms of angina pectoris
- Positive exercise ECG
- Normal coronary arteries at coronary angiography.
  Possible causes are:
- coronary artery spasm
- microvascular abnormalities.

The treatment for this syndrome is nitrates and calcium channel antagonists; the prognosis is good.

MANAGEMENT OF ANGINA PECTORIS

Management of angina involves two areas that are addressed simultaneously:

1. Management of any modifiable risk factors.
2. Management of the angina itself.

Management of the risk factors

- Ban smoking. Patients who smoke should – at all stages of management – be actively discouraged. All health professionals should be involved, and positive encouragement, advice on the complications of smoking and information about self-help groups should all be made available to smokers. Smoking-cessation clinics (which often work on a self-referral basis) are now commonplace.
- Hypertension should be diagnosed. Lifestyle modifications are important (weight loss, reduced dietary sodium intake and increased physical activity). Medications (often multiple) may be needed to bring the BP into the desired range (<140/<80). Regular monitoring is required to ensure that targets are met and maintained.
- Diabetes mellitus – blood glucose levels should be tightly controlled, by careful dietary control, oral medications and or injected insulin.
- Hypercholesterolaemia should also be treated (Fig. 9.3). Some centres recommend that patients who have coronary artery disease should have total cholesterol maintained under 5 mmol/L with low-density lipoprotein (LDL) maintained below 3 mmol/L. Others centres have slightly higher or lower recommended levels. Diet therapy should be tried first, but it is vital that, after a fixed period of dietary modification (e.g. 3 months), the fasting lipid profile is checked again and pharmacological agents used if the target levels have not been attained. The trials mentioned in Fig. 9.2 should be read because they have dramatically altered the way hypercholesterolaemia is treated.

Treatment of the angina

Drug therapy

The main drugs used in the treatment of angina are aspirin, β-blockers (β-adrenoceptor antagonists), calcium channel antagonists, nitrates and potassium channel openers.

Fig. 9.3a Drugs used to treat hypercholesterolaemia

Drug	Notes	Examples	Action	Indication	Adverse effects	Information from clinical trials
HMG CoA reductase inhibitors	Mainstay of treatment; generally well tolerated and effective; taken only once daily	Simvastatin, pravastatin, atorvastatin, fluvastatin, rosuvastatin	Inhibition of HMG CoA reductase, the rate-limiting intrahepatic enzyme in cholesterol synthesis; intracellular cholesterol levels fall leading to upregulation of apolipoprotein B and E receptors on the cell surface, resulting in increased clearance of these from the blood; LDL cholesterol levels fall	Most effective cholesterol-lowering agents available and so first-line therapy	Hepatotoxicity (LFTs should be checked before therapy and then 6-monthly); myositis – patients may complain of muscle tenderness (creatine kinase should be checked and if significantly elevated the agent should be discontinued)	Many studies show that statins reduce cardiovascular mortality of patients who have and do not have a previous history of coronary artery disease (e.g. SSSS, CARE, WOSCOPS and LIPID studies)
Fibric acid derivatives	Also reduce fibrinogen	Clofibrate, gemfibrozil, fenofibrate	Increased lipoprotein lipase activity leading to decreased VLDL; there is a significant reduction in the blood triglyceride levels and a less significant decrease in blood cholesterol concentration; there is also reduced platelet aggregation	If statins not tolerated or contraindicated or severe hypertriglycerid-aemia	Non-specific gastrointestinal symptoms; occasional myositis, especially if combined with a statin	Helsinki Heart Study showed that, when compared with placebo, gemfibrozil reduced cardiovascular mortality in hypercholesterol-aemic men at 5-year follow-up
Bile acid sequestrants		Colestyramine	Interrupt enterohepatic recycling of bile acids by binding them in the gut from where they are excreted in the faeces; bile acid synthesis increases, resulting in decreased intracellular cholesterol and therefore upregulation of apolipoprotein B and E receptors	Some familial hyperlipidaemias	Gastrointestinal (e.g. reflux, nausea)	Reduces lipids, but no mortality rate data

CAD, coronary artery disease; HMG CoA, 3-hydroxy-3-methylglutaryl coenzyme A; LDL, low-density lipoprotein; LFTs, liver function tests; SSSS, Scandinavian Simvastatin Survival Study; VLDL, very low-density lipoprotein.

Fig. 9.3b Drugs used to treat hypercholesterolaemia – Cont'd

Drug	Notes	Examples	Action	Indication	Adverse effects	Information from clinical trials
Ezetimibe				Adjust to statins	Abdominal pain, diarrhoea impairment	
Nicotinic acid	Rarely tolerated			Some familial hyperlipidaemias	Flushing, dizziness, headache, palpitations, pruritus, nausea, vomiting, impaired liver function, rashes	
Vitamin E	Normal vitamin				None in μg or mg doses	Ongoing
Fish oil	Normal component of diet	Maxepa omega 3			Nausea, belching	Ongoing
Folic acid	Normal vitamin				None	Ongoing

Aspirin

Aspirin acts to reduce platelet aggregation, which is a risk factor for the development and progression of atherosclerotic plaques.

β-Blockers

These agents are negatively inotropic and chronotropic and, therefore, reduce myocardial oxygen demand; swinging the balance of demand and supply. They are also effective antihypertensive agents and in some patients can perform a dual role reducing the need for multiple drug therapy. Remember that β-blockers are contraindicated in:

- unstable cardiac failure
- asthma
- peripheral vascular disease – a relative contraindication as the more $β_1$-selective agents may be used (e.g. bisoprolol).

Other side effects include:

- nightmares – use a non-fat-soluble agent (e.g. atenolol)
- loss of sympathetic response to hypoglycaemia – use a more cardioselective agent
- male impotence
- postural hypotension – especially in elderly patients who should start on a small dose initially.

Calcium channel antagonists

The slowing of calcium influx to the myocardial cells results in a negative inotropic response. The blockade of calcium channels in peripheral arteries results in relaxation and, therefore, vasodilatation. This improves blood flow. The blockade of calcium channels in the atrioventricular node increases the refractory period and, therefore, slows the heart rate. Agents in this group have actions on one or more of these areas and this affects the way they should be used:

- Nifedipine – dilates both coronary and peripheral vessels and can be used as an antihypertensive and antianginal drug. Main side effects are flushing, reflex tachycardia and ankle oedema

- Diltiazem – dilates coronary arteries and has some negative inotropic and chronotropic effects. It is, therefore, a good antianginal drug. It has less effect on peripheral vessels. It causes less flushing and oedema and no reflex tachycardia
- Verapamil – has almost no peripheral effects; its main effects are on the atrioventricular node and myocardium. It can, therefore, be used as an antianginal agent, but is used mainly as an antiarrhythmic
- Amlodipine – a long-acting agent with actions similar to those of nifedipine. It is an effective antianginal and antihypertensive agent.

Nitrates

These act by conversion to nitric oxide, which is a potent vasodilator (so mimicking the endothelial release of nitric oxide). The vasodilatation affects:

- veins – shifting blood from the central compartment (heart, pulmonary vessels) to peripheral veins
- arteries – reducing arterial pressure
- coronary arteries – improving myocardial perfusion.

There are a variety of preparations:

- Sublingual – glyceryl trinitrate or isosorbide dinitrate can both be taken sublingually from where they are absorbed and rapidly enter the blood. There is no risk of tolerance. Glyceryl trinitrate tablets should be changed every 6 months because they have a short shelf-life. Sublingual sprays do not have this problem.
- Transdermal – these take the form of patches or cream that allows the drug to be absorbed through the skin. Care should be taken to vary the location of the application each day.
- Oral nitrates – these may be once, twice or three times a day dosages.

Potassium channel openers

There are many families of potassium channels found in cardiac and vascular smooth muscle, and these are still incompletely understood. Nicorandil is a potassium channel opener that has been increasingly used to treat angina. The action of potassium channel openers results in venous and arterial dilatation (coronary and systemic). Potassium channel openers also act to precondition the myocardium against ischaemia, so limiting the area of myocardium vulnerable to ischaemia.

Side effects of potassium channel openers are similar to those of nitrates (i.e. headache and flushing). Tolerance is not a problem.

Management plan for angina pectoris

A possible plan of action is, therefore, the following:

- Prescribe all patients aspirin
- Prescribe a β-blocker if not contraindicated
- If β-blockade fails to control the symptoms or is contraindicated, there is a choice to start either a calcium antagonist, and be prepared to add a long-acting nitrate, or nicorandil, if the effect is still insufficient, or to prescribe nicorandil, which has effects similar to those produced by a combination of calcium antagonist and nitrate.

When diagnosing ischaemia, remember that:

- angina patients have additional ischaemic episodes that do not cause pain. These are called 'silent ischaemia' and are detectable on Holter monitoring
- silent ischaemia is more common in diabetics who have autonomic neuropathy
- drug therapy needs to be tailored to the characteristics of the individual patient.

Revascularization

There are two main ways of improving myocardial blood supply and coronary angiography is required to make the judgement:

1. Percutaneous intervention (PCI), which consists of both percutaneous transluminal coronary angioplasty (PTCA), which forces the lumen open by means of an inflated intraluminal balloon, and intracoronary stent implantation
2. Coronary artery bypass grafting (CABG).

Percutaneous intervention

PCI achieves revascularization by the inflation of a small balloon placed across a stenotic lesion;

following balloon dilatation of the stenosis a balloon mounted intracoronary stent is implanted. The procedure is carried out in the catheter laboratory under local anaesthetic and light sedation. A guide-wire is passed into the aorta via the femoral or radial artery and the balloon catheter is passed over it. Once the balloon catheter has been positioned across the stenotic plaque to be treated the balloon is inflated.

Advantages of percutaneous transluminal coronary angioplasty

The advantages of this technique over CABG are as follows:

- The patient avoids major surgery, general anaesthesia and cardiopulmonary bypass.
- There is a shortened hospital stay compared with CABG.
- Patients who have clotting disorders or who have recently had thrombolysis can be treated in an emergency.
- If PTCA is unsuccessful, CABG can still be performed (whereas a second CABG operation carries a much higher risk).

Disadvantages of PTCA

- Not all patients will have coronary artery disease that is amenable to PCI. Patients with complex coronary disease, such as stenosis of the left main stem, multi-vessel disease and chronically occluded vessels may be better served by CABG.

- Approximately 10% of patients who have had PCI will develop 'in-stent restenosis' (ISR). This rate is higher in diabetic patients, and those that have long segments of stent and smaller calibre stents. ISR can be treated by further PCI. The rate of ISR has been reduced by the introduction of stents coated with drugs that inhibit the endothelial response to stent implantation; these are known as drug eluting stents (DES). DES are significantly more expensive than their bare metal counterparts and, thus, in the UK their use is rationed to patients who are deemed at the highest risk of ISR.
- Thrombosis at the site of stenting may occur and is partly prevented by the rigorous use of intravenous heparin at the time of PCI, and long-term oral antiplatelet aggregation agents (Fig. 9.4).

Complications of percutaneous transluminal coronary angioplasty

These include major adverse effects such as:

- myocardial infarction – secondary to thrombosis, spasm of the coronary artery, or dissection of the coronary artery by the balloon
- coronary artery perforation
- stroke
- less severe, but more common adverse effects such as:
  - ○ arrhythmias
  - ○ dye reactions (allergy and nephrotoxicity)
  - ○ haemorrhage or infection at the puncture site.

Fig. 9.4 Antiplatelet agents used to prevent thrombosis following PTCA ± stenting

Class of drug and examples	Action	Side-effects
NSAIDs (e.g. aspirin)	Irreversible inactivation of cyclooxygenase – within platelets this enzyme is needed for the production of thromboxane (a stimulator of platelet aggregation)	Gastritis (possibly with ulcer formation and bleeding), renal impairment, bronchospasm, rashes
Platelet ADP receptor antagonists (e.g. clopidogrel)	When activated the adenyl cyclase-coupled ADP receptor causes binding of fibrinogen to the platelet and initiation of thrombus formation – this is irreversibly inhibited by these agents	Haemorrhage, diarrhoea, nausea, neutropenia, hepatic dysfunction
Platelet membrane glycoprotein IIb/IIIa receptor inhibitors (abciximab is a monoclonal antibody that binds to and blocks this receptor)	The GP IIa/IIIb platelet receptor binds fibrinogen, von Willebrand's factor and other adhesive molecules – blockade therefore inhibits platelet aggregation and thrombus formation	Haemorrhage

ADP, adenosine diphosphate; NSAIDs, non-steroidal anti-inflammatory drugs.

Coronary artery bypass grafting

CAGB aims to achieve revascularization by bypassing a stenotic lesion using grafts.

The patient undergoes a full general anaesthetic and the heart is exposed via a median sternotomy.

Cardiopulmonary bypass is achieved by inserting a cannula into the right atrium and another into the proximal aorta. The two cannulas are connected to the bypass machine, which oxygenates the venous blood from the right atrium and feeds it back to the aorta.

The heart is stopped using cooling and cardioplegic solutions.

Vein grafts harvested from the great saphenous vein or arterial grafts are used to bypass the occlusive coronary lesions.

Arterial grafts are preferred given that they have much better long-term patency than vein grafts. The arteries commonly used for grafting include the left and right internal mammary arteries, and to a lesser extent the radial arteries.

Complications of coronary artery bypass grafting

These are:

- death – mortality rates are approximately 1%
- myocardial infarction, stroke and peripheral thromboembolism
- wound infection
- complications related to cardiopulmonary bypass – these are related to the haemodilution involved and the exposure of the blood to synthetic materials in the oxygenating process; they include clotting and pulmonary abnormalities, and impaired cognitive function.

Minimally invasive coronary artery bypass grafting

Minimally invasive CABG (MICABG) is a new technique that involves a smaller incision, usually a left anterior minithoracotomy. The left or right internal mammary artery is used to graft the occluded vessel (usually the left anterior descending coronary artery because this is situated within easy reach). Cardiopulmonary bypass is not used – instead the heart is slowed using β-blockers and a specifically designed instrument is used to immobilize the small area around the anastomosis.

UNSTABLE ANGINA

This condition is one of the acute coronary syndromes. The pathophysiology underlying unstable angina involves rupture of an atherosclerotic plaque within the coronary artery and the subsequent formation of a thrombus over this. The result is a rapid reduction in the size of the lumen of the vessel.

Clinically, unstable angina is defined as:

- new onset (<6 weeks) angina at exertion or at rest
- angina at rest in previously exercise-induced angina
- exertional angina that is not responding to increasing antianginal medications.

Plasma troponin levels (troponin T or troponin I) are now being determined routinely. A significantly raised troponin level suggests myocardial necrosis and the patient is then said to have sustained a myocardial infarction rather than unstable angina.

Management

The following management plan should be followed:

- Admit the patient to the coronary care unit for observation and strict bed rest – remember that if the thrombus extends and completely occludes the vessel lumen a myocardial infarction will occur.
- Provide analgesia with intravenous diamorphine (2.5–5 mg intravenously) if required to calm the patient and relieve pain – remember to give metoclopramide too.
- Give aspirin – it has been shown to reduce the incidence of myocardial infarction and death in patients who have unstable angina (300 mg soluble aspirin).
- Give clopidogrel (300 mg loading dose) followed by 75 mg OD. This has been shown to reduce mortality in acute coronary syndrome.
- Give an intravenous infusion of nitrates (e.g. glyceryl trinitrate 0.5–10 mg/h) to dilate the coronary arteries and reduce the load on the heart by peripheral vasodilatation and venodilatation. The blood pressure will drop so it should be carefully monitored.
- Give low-molecular-weight heparin (LMWH) (or unfractionated heparin as a 24-h infusion)

to prevent further thrombus formation. LMWHs are given at doses according to patient weight and no such measurements are required. There is evidence to suggest that the LMWHs are more effective than intravenous heparin. Intravenous heparin has the disadvantage that the activated partial thromboplastin time needs to be monitored to ensure that it does not become too high and lead to haemorrhage

- Once the patient is more stable start oral antianginal therapy and arrange early angiography if appropriate.

Heparins

Heparin comprises a highly heterogeneous group of compounds – all are proteoglycans, but they differ in their constituent sugar units and in their molecular weight.

Heparin acts to alter antithrombin, which becomes much more effective in inhibiting thrombin and the coagulation factors Xa and IXa.

The problems with heparin administration for unstable angina are as follows:

- To maintain a constant effect heparin must be given as an intravenous infusion. Therefore, the patient must be an inpatient and be relatively immobile.
- During this time the activated partial thromboplastin time must be regularly monitored to ensure that the effect of heparin is not too little (rendering the drug ineffective) or too great (leading to a risk of haemorrhage).

Side effects of heparin include osteoporosis and thrombocytopenia.

LMWHs form a more uniform group of heparins with 13–22 sugar residues. They have high bioavailability after subcutaneous injection and a longer half-life. They also have a more predictable anticoagulant effect than conventional heparin. The benefits of LMWHs are:

- they can be given as twice daily subcutaneous injections instead of as a continuous infusion
- the dose is adjusted according to patient weight and the anticoagulant effect is sufficiently predictable that regular monitoring is not required
- there is a lower risk of osteoporosis and thrombocytopenia.

Further reading

Antithrombotic Trialists' Collaboration 2002 Collaborative meta-analysis of randomised trials of antiplatelet therapy for prevention of death, myocardial infarction, and stroke in high risk patients. *BMJ* **324**: 71–86

Braunwald E, Antman E M, Beasley J W et al 2002 ACC/AHA 2002 guideline update for the management of patients with unstable angina and non-ST-segment elevation myocardial infarction: a report of the American College of Cardiology/ American Heart Association task force on practice. *J Am Coll Cardiol* **40**: 1366–74

Cannon C P, Braunwald E 2001 'Unstable Angina'. In: Braunwald E, Zipes D P (eds) Heart Disease: A Textbook of Cardiovascular Medicine, 6th edn. W B Saunders & Co

The Clopidogrel in Unstable Angina to Prevent Recurrent Events Trial Investigators August 2001 Effects of clopidogrel in addition to aspirin in patients with acute coronary syndromes without ST-segment elevation. *N Engl J Med* **345**: 494–502

Grech E D, Ramsdale D R June 2003 Acute coronary syndrome: unstable angina and non-ST segment elevation myocardial infarction. *BMJ* **326**: 1259–61

Knopp R H 1999 Drug treatment of lipid disorders. *N Engl J Med* **341**: 498–511

Lee T H 2001 Guidelines: management of unstable angina/non-ST segment elevation myocardial infarction. In: Braunwald E, Zipes D P (eds) Heart Disease: A Textbook of Cardiovascular Medicine, 6th edn. W B Saunders & Co

Acute myocardial infarction

Objectives

By the end of this chapter you should:

- be able to describe the temporal changes of the various cardiac biomarkers after myocardial infarction
- be able to recognize the common cardiac complications that occur in the first 48 h following acute myocardial infarction and understand their management
- understand the common cardiac complications that occur in the first 7 days following acute myocardial infarction
- understand the emergency management for patients presenting with acute myocardial infarction
- understand the different revascularization strategies available to treat acute myocardial infarction.

DEFINITION OF ACUTE MYOCARDIAL INFARCTION

Acute myocardial infarction (MI) is the term used for cell death secondary to ischaemia. The most common cause of MI is atherosclerotic narrowing of the coronary arteries. The immediate precursor to MI is rupture of an atherosclerotic plaque and the formation of thrombus over the plaque resulting in rapid occlusion of the vessel.

Traditionally acute MI has been defined according to the 1971 World Health Organization criteria based on the presence of at least two of clinical syndrome, ECG changes and elevations in relatively non-specific markers of myocardial damage such as creatine kinase. This definition has recently been updated to include cardiac troponins as a more sensitive and specific biomarker for myocardial necrosis (Fig. 10.1).

Depending on the rate of vessel occlusion (if an atherosclerotic plaque grows slowly, over months, collateral vessels develop and protect the myocardium) and the degree of occlusion of the vessel by thrombus, a number of clinical conditions can result from plaque rupture. These conditions are termed the acute coronary syndromes. Acute MI is the most serious of this spectrum of acute illnesses (Fig. 10.2).

For simplicity, and to make the management algorithm work (see below), these are divided into two categories:

1. ST elevation
2. no ST elevation.

All these syndromes present as severe central chest pain of typical cardiac type (see Ch. 1) and patients usually present at the accident and emergency department with one of the following:

- Severe angina – there is a history of angina and the pain usually subsides spontaneously with rest and nitrates without permanent change to the ECG or evidence of activation of coagulation or myocardial damage.
- A sudden increase in exertional angina – there is rupture of an atheromatous plaque in the coronary artery, which causes a step decrease in its luminal diameter; the pain usually subsides spontaneously with rest and nitrates, without permanent change to the ECG or evidence of activation of coagulation or myocardial damage. The condition may progress to full infarction.
- Widespread subendocardial ischaemia – ST depression may be present in all ECG leads except AVR. This is a manifestation of critical stenoses in all three coronary arteries.

Fig. 10.1 Joint European Society of Cardiology/American College of Cardiology criteria

Criteria for acute, evolving, or recent myocardial infarction (MI) – one of the following:

1. Typical rise and fall of biochemical markers of myocardial necrosis with at least one of the following:
   a. ischaemic symptoms
   b. Q waves
   c. ischaemic ECG changes
   d. coronary artery intervention
2. Pathological findings of an acute MI

Criteria for established MI – any of the following:

1. Development of new pathological Q waves on serial ECGs
2. Pathological findings of a healed or healing MI

Fig. 10.2 Acute coronary syndromes in order of severity (↑)

Q wave infarction
Non-Q wave infarction
Unstable angina due to coronary arterial thrombosis
Widespread subendocardial ischaemia
Sudden increase in severity of exertional angina
Severe angina episode in a patient who has exertional angina

There is no evidence of activation of coagulation or myocardial damage, but the prognosis is very poor without emergency treatment.

- Unstable angina due to coronary arterial thrombosis – there is no ST elevation, but microinfarcts may be occurring due to embolization of thrombi from the site of plaque rupture downstream.
- Non-Q-wave infarction – this is necrosis caused by thrombotic coronary artery occlusion in which the myocardial cell death is confined to the endocardial layers and is not full thickness. It occurs because the occluded artery is a relatively small branch, because there is good collateral flow around the occluded vessel or because thrombolysis for ST elevation has been early and effective.
- Q-wave infarction – this follows necrosis through the whole thickness of the ventricular wall, leaving permanent Q waves on the ECG (Fig. 10.3).

CLINICAL FEATURES OF ACUTE MYOCARDIAL INFARCTION

History

The history is very important because it provides clues about the severity of the infarction and the time of onset (important when deciding on therapy). The following are classic features of the history of acute MI.

Presenting complaint

The main presenting complaint is of chest pain. The following characteristics are common:

- Usually severe in nature
- Normally lasts at least 30 min
- Usually tight, crushing and bandlike in nature
- Retrosternal in location
- May radiate to the left arm, throat or jaw
- Associated features include sweating, breathlessness and nausea.

Elderly patients may have relatively little pain, but present with features of left ventricular failure (profound breathlessness) or syncope.

Past medical history

Important features include a history of angina or intermittent chest pain that often increases in severity or frequency in the few weeks preceding this event.

Risk factors for ischaemic heart disease are smoking, hypertension, diabetes mellitus, hypercholesterolaemia and positive family history. (Although some of these do not belong in this section of the clerking, it is important not to forget these and, therefore, easier to ask about them all together at the same time.)

The patient may have a history of previous MI or of cardiac intervention, such as angiography, percutaneous transluminal coronary angioplasty (PTCA) or CABG.

Also ask about any contraindication for thrombolysis at this stage (see p. 83).

Examination

On inspection, the patient is often extremely anxious and distressed and will often be restless; he or she may be in severe pain. Breathlessness suggests the presence of pulmonary oedema, as does the presence of pink frothy sputum. The patient may be pale, clammy and sweaty, suggesting a degree of cardiogenic shock. Look for scars of previous surgery.

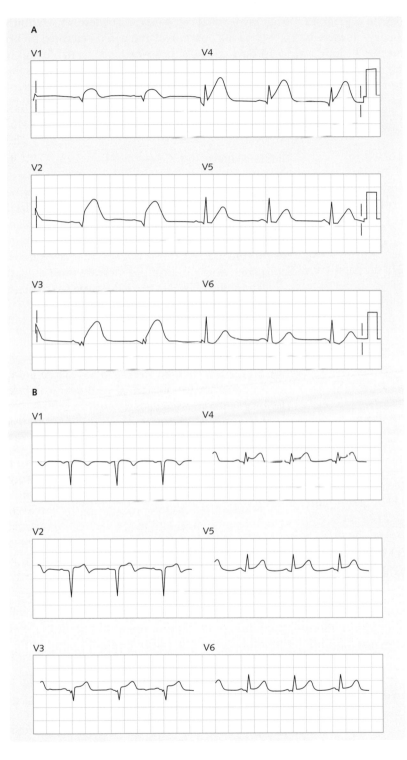

Fig. 10.3 (A) ECG showing acute anterior myocardial infarction (MI). (B) ECG 24 h after anterior MI. Note the resolution of the ST elevation and the development of Q waves. The loss of the R wave in this ECG suggests that a significant left-ventricle muscle mass has undergone necrosis.

Cardiovascular system

The pulse may be tachycardic secondary to anxiety or left ventricular failure, or it may be bradycardic in the case of an inferior MI where the right coronary artery is occluded and the atrioventricular node (which is supplied by the right coronary artery in 90% of people) is affected.

Although the blood pressure may be normal, in some patients it is raised due to anxiety. If there is cardiogenic shock the blood pressure may be low.

The jugular venous pressure may be elevated in cases of congestive cardiac failure or in pure right-ventricular infarction.

Examination of the praecordium may reveal the following:

- A displaced diffuse apex in cases of left ventricular failure.
- In anterior infarction a paradoxical systolic outward movement of the ventricular wall may be felt parasternally.
- Audible murmurs.
- The murmur of mitral regurgitation – may occur as a new murmur due to rupture of the papillary muscle.
- A pericardial rub – may be audible in some patients because it is not uncommon for an MI to be complicated by pericarditis.
- A fourth heart sound (Fig. 10.4) – common in MI due to reduction of left-ventricular compliance.
- A third heart sound – occurs in the presence of left ventricular failure.
- Further evidence of cardiac failure (e.g. bilateral basal crepitations, peripheral oedema and poor peripheral perfusion).

INVESTIGATION OF ACUTE MYOCARDIAL INFARCTION

Blood tests

Indicators of myocardial damage

Troponin T and troponin I

Troponin T and troponin I are proteins that form part of the myocardial cell structure. Release of these proteins into the bloodstream indicates that there has been myocardial cell damage. The levels rise within 6–14 h of the onset of MI and remain elevated for up to 14 days. This test is now widely available and is used in both diagnosis and risk stratification, as the increase in cardiac troponin is related to the risk of cardiac complications. Troponin increase should be regarded as only one of the independent predictors of risk in patients with ACS.

Creatine kinase

The MB isoenzyme of creatine kinase (CK) increases and falls within 72 h. The source of CK-MB isoenzyme is cardiac muscle, whereas CK-MM is found in skeletal muscle and CK-BB is in brain and kidney. Many laboratories provide only total CK measurements for routine use and this is not specific. The CK-MB isoenzyme does not begin to increase until at least 4 h after infarction and is, therefore, not used to make the initial diagnosis in most cases.

Renal function and electrolytes

These are important in all patients who have MI. Renal function may be deranged or may worsen due to poor renal perfusion in cardiogenic shock. Hypokalaemia may predispose to arrhythmias and must be corrected because acute MI is in itself a proarrhythmogenic condition.

Blood glucose

Diabetes mellitus must be controlled aggressively after MI and all patients who have diabetes mellitus benefit from insulin therapy either using an intravenous sliding scale or, if stable, four times daily subcutaneous insulin.

Full blood count

Anaemia may precipitate an acute MI in a patient who has angina. There is often a leucocytosis after acute MI.

Fig. 10.4 Notes on third and fourth heart sounds

Heart sound	Mechanism	When heard	Causes
Fourth	Represents atrial contribution to ventricular filling	Heard in any condition that causes a 'stiff' left ventricular wall	Hypertension, aortic stenosis, acute MI
Third	Rapid filling of the ventricle as soon as the mitral valve opens	Normal finding in the young and heard in conditions where there is fluid overload of the ventricle	Mitral regurgitation, ventricular septal defect, left ventricular failure, MI

MI, myocardial infarction.

Serum cholesterol

This should be measured within 24 h of an MI; hypercholesterolaemia is a risk factor for MI and needs to be treated. Cholesterol level falls to an artificially low level 24 h after MI, so after this time a true reading can only be obtained 2 months after MI.

Electrocardiography

The ECG is the main diagnostic test in acute MI (Fig. 10.5) and it is, therefore, important to have a thorough knowledge of the ECG appearances of different types of MI. Delay in the diagnosis wastes precious time because thrombolysis should be given as soon as possible for maximum benefit.

Classic ECG changes of a full-thickness MI are as follows:

- ST segment elevation – this is due to full-thickness myocardial injury and may appear within minutes of the onset of infarction; it is almost always present by 24 h. The criteria for acute thrombolysis are a good history and ST segment elevation greater than 1 mm in two or more consecutive leads. Reciprocal ST segment depression may be present at the same time and represents the mirror image of the ST elevation as seen from the opposite side of the heart.
- Over 24 h the ST elevation resolves and the T waves begin to invert.
- Q waves develop within 24–72 h of MI.

Persistent elevation of ST segments after 1 week indicates either reinfarction or a left-ventricular aneurysm.

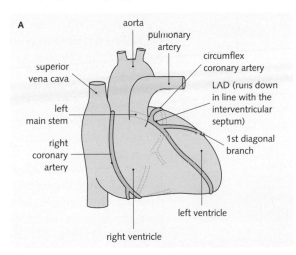

Fig. 10.5 (A) Location of coronary arteries. Note the left anterior descending coronary artery branch (LAD) supplies the anterior aspect of the heart (the left ventricle and the septum), the right coronary artery (RCA) supplies the inferoposterior aspect and the circumflex supplies the lateral part of the left ventricle. (B) ST elevation in leads I, AVL and V4–6.

Fig. 10.5B ST elevation in leads

Location of MI	ECG changes
Anterior (LAD)	ST elevation in leads V1–4
Inferior (RCA or circumflex coronary artery)	ST elevation in leads II, III, AVF
Lateral (circumflex coronary artery)	ST elevation in leads V4–6
Posterior (RCA or circumflex coronary artery)	Prominent R wave in V1 and V2 with ST depression (mirror image of anterior MI)
Anterolateral (proximal LAD) above diagonal branch	ST elevation V1–6
Right ventricular infarction (suspect in inferior or posterior MI)	Perform right-sided ECG using lead V1 (as normal), leads V3–6 placed on the right side, limb leads as normal

ECG changes in non-Q-wave myocardial infarction

These are variable and the absence of Q waves does not necessarily indicate that full-thickness infarction has not occurred. The conventional view used to be that this represented subendocardial damage only.

The ECG changes tend to be in the form of persistent T wave inversion accompanied by an increase in cardiac enzymes.

Chest radiography

This should be performed on all patients who have acute MI. Points to note are:

- widening of the mediastinum – suggests a likelihood of aortic dissection, which is an absolute contraindication for thrombolysis
- signs of pulmonary oedema – signify the need for antifailure therapy (intravenous diuretics, oxygen and possibly a nitrate infusion)
- an enlarged heart – suggests cardiac failure.

Echocardiography

This is not a first-line investigation, but is very useful in the first week to assess left-ventricular function or investigate valve lesions (mitral regurgitation may occur after MI as a result of papillary muscle infarction).

MANAGEMENT OF ACUTE MYOCARDIAL INFARCTION

Acute MI is a medical emergency and, therefore, you must know its acute management thoroughly (Fig. 10.6). It is one of the few occasions in an examination when you will be expected to know the doses of drugs given.

In the context of cardiac chest pain, ST segment elevation on the 12-lead ECG usually signifies complete occlusion of a proximal epicardial coronary artery. If untreated myocardial necrosis commences within 30 min, affecting full myocardial thickness within 6 h. Forty per cent of patients die before reaching hospital.

Treatment

Urgent restoration of coronary blood flow (reperfusion) prevents further left-ventricular damage and improves prognosis. The amount of myocardium that can be salvaged falls exponentially with time, the greatest benefit being within 3 h of symptom onset, and little benefit after 12 h.

Options for reperfusion include the following:

- Primary angioplasty – primary angioplasty is the preferred reperfusion strategy if an angiogram can be performed within 90 min of presentation. This service is still not yet widely available in the UK and such treatment is usually reserved for patients presenting to hospitals with an on-site angioplasty service.
- Thrombolysis – a number of large, prospective, double-blind, placebo-controlled trials have shown that thrombolysis reduces mortality rate after MI, for example the Italian GISSI trial and the International Study of Infarct Survival (ISIS) 2 study. This is because thrombolysis results in recanalization of the occluded vessel and restores coronary flow, which reduces infarct size and improves myocardial function if thrombolysis is administered within 24 h of pain.

Thrombolytic agents

There are a number of thrombolytic agents (Fig. 10.7). The two most commonly used are streptokinase and

---

Fig. 10.6 Acute management of acute myocardial infarction

- Administer oxygen via a facial mask
- Give the patient soluble aspirin 300 mg in water
- Establish IV access and connect patient to cardiac monitor
- If patient is distressed or in pain give diamorphine 2.5–5 mg IV with 10 mg metoclopramide
- If patient satisfies the criteria for thrombolysis and has no contraindications administer thrombolysis: streptokinase 1.5 million units in 100 mL normal saline IV over 1 hour or rt-PA if the patient has ever had streptokinase before or is young (<65) and has an anterior MI
- Administer intravenous atenolol 5 mg over 10 min; if tolerated, repeat the dose after 10 min
- Continue to observe the patient in the coronary care unit

IV, intravenous; rt-PA, recombinant tissue plasminogen activator.

Fig. 10.7 Overview of thrombolytic agents

Agent	Action	Half-life (min)	Administration	Other features
Streptokinase	Binds to plasminogen to form a complex that activates to convert another molecule of plasminogen to plasmin; not clot specific – will attack all plasminogen	18 (but 180 for streptokinase plasminogen complex)	Infusion of 1.5 million units over 1 h	Allergic reactions, hypotension, previous streptokinase treatment renders subsequent doses less effective due to antibody production, haemorrhage
rt-PA (Alteplase)	Binds to fibrin and complex converts plasminogen to plasmin; clot specific – will act only in presence of fibrin	4–5 (circulating plasminogen and fibrinogen levels return to 80% of normal within 24 h)	Infusion, often preceded by a bolus dose; accelerated rt-PA – 15-mg bolus then 50 mg over 30 min followed by 35 mg over 1 h (as in the GUSTO trial)	Haemorrhage, expensive
Reteplase	Same as Alteplase		2 bolus injections 30 minutes apart	
Tenecteplase	Same as Alteplase		500–600 micrograms/kg Single bolus injection	
The ideal thrombolytic agent	Very clot specific, easily reversible in the event of haemorrhage; administration by intravenous bolus	Very short half-life for use in hospital as infusion (can be easily controlled) and long half-life preparation for community use where coronary care not easily accessible		Cheap, no antibody effects, derived from human protein so no anaphylaxis

APSAC, anisoylated plasminogen-streptokinase activator complex; GUSTO, Global Use of Strategies to Open Occluded Arteries; IV, intravenous; rt-PA, recombinant tissue plasminogen activator.

recombinant tissue plasminogen activator (rt-PA). There are, however, an increasing number of new agents.

Two major trials – GISSI II and ISIS 3 – showed no increased benefit when comparing different thrombolytic agents (GISSI II: streptokinase and t-PA; ISIS 3: streptokinase, rt-PA and anisoylated plasminogen-streptokinase activator complex (APSAC)). These trials also showed that heparin provided no benefit. However, the GUSTO (Global Use of Strategies to Open Occluded Arteries) 1 trial showed a small benefit with accelerated rt-PA followed by a heparin infusion over other regimens.

Contraindications to thrombolysis

All final-year students and junior doctors must know this list:

- History of haemorrhagic cerebrovascular event – ever
- History of any type of cerebrovascular event – in the past 6 months
- Recent gastrointestinal bleed
- Bleeding diathesis
- Operation within past month – not an absolute contraindication, but you should consult a senior before proceeding

- Pregnancy
- Any other invasive procedure in the past month (e.g. organ biopsy, dental extraction) – consult a senior before proceeding.

Indications for thrombolysis

Most centres consider a door-to-needle time of greater than 30 min unacceptable. If they are to receive the greatest benefit, patients should be thrombolysed within 70 min of the onset of pain. All patients who satisfy the following criteria should be thrombolysed as soon as possible:

- History of chest pain lasting less than 24 h
- One of the following – ST elevation >1 mm in standard leads or in two adjacent chest leads, new bundle branch block on ECG

Other agents used for acute myocardial infarction

Aspirin

The antiplatelet aggregation action of aspirin makes it effective in all acute coronary syndromes where the primary event is clot formation. This drug has relatively few side effects and should be administered promptly to all patients as soon as the ECG is found to be positive. Aspirin was found to reduce the mortality rate in the ISIS 2 study.

Diamorphine

A powerful anxiolytic and analgesic, this drug is extremely effective in patients with cardiac pain. It has venodilating properties and is, therefore, also an effective antifailure agent.

β-Blockers (β-adrenoceptor antagonists)

These drugs were shown to reduce mortality rate acutely after MI in the ISIS 1 study. The following are contraindications to the administration of β-blockers:

- Unstable or acute cardiac failure
- Bradycardia (heart rate <60 beats/min)
- Hypotension (systolic blood pressure <90 mmHg)
- Asthma.

Oxygen

Oxygen should be administered to all patients initially and then continued for all patients who have hypoxaemia (i.e. arterial oxygen saturation 90%).

Non-acute management

The first 5–7 days after MI are spent in hospital because this is when most complications (Fig. 10.8) will arise.

The following points of management must be observed. The patient must be seen and examined every day by a cardiologist. Particular points to look for on examination and questioning are:

- chest pain – further pain indicates the possibility of another MI and should be investigated early with urgent coronary angiography
- breathlessness or signs of cardiac failure – diuretics should be commenced and urgent echocardiography performed to exclude septal defect or mitral regurgitation secondary to papillary muscle rupture
- new murmurs – a ruptured papillary muscle causes mitral regurgitation; a ruptured septum causes ventricular septal defect
- pericardial rub – pericarditis
- hypotension – drug induced or secondary to cardiogenic shock
- bradycardia – heart block after an inferior MI (or very large anterior MI with septal necrosis).

Patients should have daily ECGs to look for arrhythmias including heart block.

Fig. 10.8 Complications of an acute myocardial infarction

Early (0–48 h)
Arrhythmias – VT, VF, SVT, heart block
Cardiogenic shock due to left or right ventricular failure

Medium term (2–7 days)
Arrhythmias – VT,VF, SVT, heart block
Pulmonary embolus (4–7 days)
Rupture of papillary muscle (3–5 days)
Rupture of interventricular septum (3–5 days)
Free wall rupture (3–5 days)
Note: Rupture of the above structures usually presents with acute cardiac failure and progresses rapidly to death; a few patients might survive after surgery

Late (7 days)
Arrhythmias – VT, VF, SVT, heart block
Cardiac failure
Dressler's syndrome (3–8 weeks)
Left ventricular aneurysm (after several weeks)
Mural thrombosis and sytemic embolization

SVT, supraventricular tachycardia; VF, ventricular fibrillation: VT, ventricular tachycardia.

A continuous cardiac monitor should be used for the first 5 days because fatal arrhythmias are common after MI (usually ventricular tachycardia or fibrillation).

Early mobilization (after 48 h) is instituted to prevent venous stasis.

If a patient has had a large MI, or if there is clinical evidence of cardiac failure (and provided there is no renal failure or hypotension), an angiotensin-converting enzyme inhibitor should be introduced at day 3 after MI. This improves outcome (as seen in the ISIS 4 and GISSI 3 studies).

Hypercholesterolaemia should be treated with a statin and the patient referred to a lipid management clinic for follow-up. Suitable dietary advice should be given. Recent evidence suggests that a statin should be given anyway because statins may have additional benefits after MI in addition to their lipid-lowering effect. The LIPID (Long-term Intervention with Pravastatin in Ischaemic Heart Disease) study shows benefit with pravastatin in patients after MI who have total cholesterol before treatment as low as 4.0 mmol/L.

Follow-up care should include:

- an exercise test at about 6 weeks after MI to assess the risk of further ischaemia – if positive coronary angiography should be performed
- access to the rehabilitation programme.

Cardiac rehabilitation

All good cardiac units have an integrated rehabilitation programme available to all cardiac patients that consists of:

- progressively increasing exercise level to a maintenance level of as much regular rapid walking as possible every day
- dietary advice, particularly emphasizing the value of fish and olive oil, and fresh fruit and vegetables. Carbohydrate restriction for non-insulin-dependent diabetes mellitus and insulin resistance. Calorie restriction for patients who have diabetes mellitus or who are obese
- advice on medications (Fig. 10.9), their role in improving prognosis, and the importance of compliance
- advice from a clinical psychologist on how to cope with the illness

---

Fig. 10.9 Drugs on discharge after myocardial infarction

- Aspirin
- β-Blocker
- ACE inhibitor
- A statin lipid-lowering drug – should probably be given regardless of lipid levels because they seem to modify the progress of atheroma independently

ACE, angiotensin-converting enzyme.

- group gymnasium sessions may help some patients by encouraging exercise and giving psychological support to each other
- a subsequent support group may be continued as long as each individual patient finds it helpful; a doctor's input is important from time to time.

SUMMARY OF MANAGEMENT OF ISCHAEMIC CHEST PAIN

An algorithm summarizing the management of ischaemic chest pain is given in Fig. 10.10.

HEART BLOCK AFTER MYOCARDIAL INFARCTION

Ischaemic injury can occur at any point in the conducting system – the sinoatrial node, the atrioventricular node or anywhere from the bundle of His downwards. It is, therefore, not surprising that heart block after MI may be:

- first- or second-degree atrioventricular block
- complete heart block with atrioventricular dissociation
- interventricular block (complete or partial right or left bundle branch block).

Inferior MI is more commonly associated with atrioventricular block because the atrioventricular node is supplied by the right coronary artery in 90% of cases.

Anterior MI may cause heart block if there is marked septal necrosis (indicating a large anterior MI).

NODAL AND JUNCTIONAL ECTOPICS

The AV node is a compact structure and lying close to it is the AV junctional area. It is from this area and from the node itself that these ectopic beats originate. These structures have the ability to fire autonomously, but they have a slower rate of firing than the sinoatrial (SA) node; therefore, they are usually suppressed.

In some conditions, impulses arise ectopically from the AV node and junctional region. The impulse is conducted to the atrium where a retrograde P wave is produced and also to the ventricle where a narrow complex QRS is produced (Fig. 11.1). Depending on the speed of conduction, the P wave may occur just before, after or simultaneously with the QRS.

Again, treatment is not usually indicated.

ATRIAL TACHYCARDIA

Atrial tachycardia is a tachyarrhythmia generated in the atrial tissue. The atrial rate is 150–200 beats/min.

Because the origin of the tachycardia is not the SA node, the P-wave morphology is different from normal. The P wave axis may also be abnormal, for example when the atrial focus is in the left atrium the P wave in lead V1 is positive.

Causes

The following may lead to atrial tachycardia:

- Structural heart abnormality
- Coronary artery disease
- Digitalis toxicity.

Investigation and diagnosis

On examination the pulse is rapid and of variable intensity:

- Jugular venous pressure may reveal many a waves to each v wave if there is a degree of atrioventricular (AV) block.
- ECG may show 1:1 conduction or variable degrees of AV block.
- It may be difficult to differentiate atrial tachycardia from atrial flutter.

Diagnosis may be aided by enhancing AV block and, therefore, making it easier to visualize the P wave morphology and rate. There are two effective methods of doing this:

1. Carotid sinus massage – increases vagal stimulation of the SA and AV node (see p. 95)
2. Intravenous adenosine – results in transient complete AV block.

Fig. 11.1 (A) A nodal ectopic. The ectopic complex is similar to the normal QRS, suggesting that it originates from the atrioventricular or junctional region. The P wave is retrograde and is seen just after the ectopic QRS superimposed on the T wave. The ectopic beat is followed by a compensatory pause. (B) ECG illustrating an ectopic atrial beat. Note that the premature atrial beat fires an abnormally shaped P wave and a normal QRS complex. A compensatory pause follows.

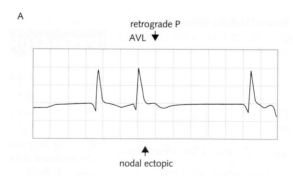

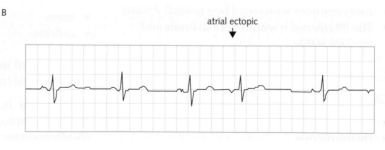

Remember that atrial flutter usually has an atrial rate of 300/min with a degree of AV block. Atrial tachycardia has a slightly slower atrial rate with abnormal P waves.

Management

The patient will present with palpitations. Any underlying cause should be treated (e.g. check digoxin levels and stop the drug).

Drugs used to treat atrial tachycardia include:

- atrioventricular blocking drugs, such as digoxin, β-blockers (β-adrenoceptor antagonists, e.g. metoprolol) and calcium channel blockers (e.g. verapamil) – these slow the ventricular response rate, but do not affect the atrial tachycardia itself
- class IA (e.g. disopyramide), IC (e.g. flecainide) or III (e.g. amiodarone) drugs (see p. 96), which can be used to try to terminate the atrial tachycardia.

Electrical cardioversion is often successful.

ATRIOVENTRICULAR JUNCTIONAL TACHYCARDIA

Tachycardias arising from the junctional area occur when there is a focus of activity with a discharge rate that is faster than that of the SA node. This is an abnormal situation and is usually due to ischaemic heart disease or digitalis toxicity.

Clinical features

The following features are seen:

- Rate is usually up to 130 beats/min
- Gradual onset
- Terminates gradually
- ECG shows a narrow complex tachycardia occasionally with retrogradely conducted P waves. It is difficult to distinguish this from an AV nodal re-entry tachycardia and you will not be expected to do so. The main point is to realize that the junctional tissue may be a site of ectopic electrical activity.

Management

Treatment is aimed at the underlying cause:

- Antiarrhythmic agents such as digoxin, β-blockers and calcium channel antagonists may be tried.
- Electrical cardioversion may be successful.

ATRIOVENTRICULAR NODAL RE-ENTRY TACHYCARDIA

These tachycardias involve a re-entry circuit that lies in or close to the AV node and allows impulses to travel round and round triggering the ventricles and the atria (in a retrograde manner) as they go.

Clinical features

These tachycardias display the following features:

- Rate is 150–260 beats/min
- Usually sudden onset and offset
- QRS complexes are narrow unless there is aberrant conduction and the P waves may occur just before, just after, or within the QRS (it is not always easy to see these; see Fig. 4.4C).

Causes of re-entry tachycardia are caffeine, alcohol and anxiety.

Diagnosis

Differentiation from atrial flutter and atrial fibrillation (AF) can be made by either:

- performing carotid sinus massage or Valsalva manoeuvre

  or

- giving intravenous adenosine.

These procedures block the AV node and, therefore, the P waves of atrial flutter can be seen or the baseline fibrillation of AF can be seen. Blockade of the AV node in re-entrant tachycardia breaks the re-entry circuit and terminates the tachycardia in most cases. Re-entry tachycardia will also be terminated by a ventricular ectopic beat.

Management

These tachycardias often terminate spontaneously with relaxation.

Fig. 12.1 Ventricular ectopic beats, which are indicated by arrows.

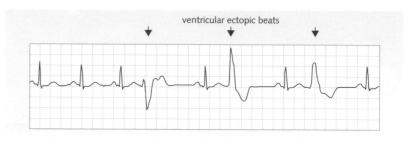

There are three basic types of ventricular tachyarrhythmia:

1. Ventricular tachycardia
2. Torsades de pointes
3. Ventricular fibrillation.

VENTRICULAR TACHYCARDIA

Ventricular tachycardia (VT) is defined as three or more consecutive ventricular beats occurring at a rate greater than 120 beats/min (Fig. 12.2). Again the complexes are abnormal and their duration is longer than 120 ms.

Clinical features

Patients may tolerate this rhythm well and experience only palpitations or rarely nothing at all. However, the reduction in cardiac output caused by this arrhythmia often causes dizziness or syncope. Common precipitants include acute MI, cardiomyopathy or inherited conduction disorders.

Diagnosis

VT may be monomorphic (complexes on the surface ECG have the same shape) or polymorphic (beat-to-beat variations in morphology). The main differential diagnosis for VT is supraventricular tachycardia

Fig. 12.2 ECG illustrating ventricular tachycardia. Note the concordance shown in the chest leads. No fusion or capture beats are visible.

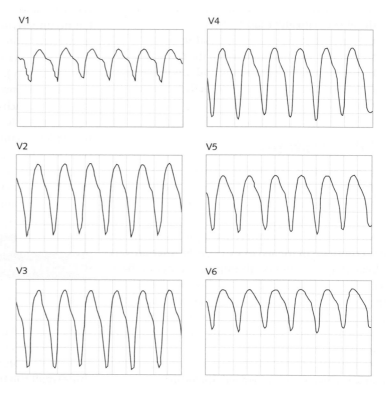

Fig. 12.3 Differences between ventricular tachycardia (VT) and supraventricular tachycardia (SVT) with bundle branch block (BBB)

Arrhythmia	VT	SVT with BBB
AV association	AV dissociation (no relationship between P waves and QRS)	P waves, if seen, are associated with the QRS
Variety of complexes	Capture beats (where a P wave is followed by a normal QRS); fusion beats (where a normal sinus beat occurs simultaneously with a ventricular beat, the resulting complex having an intermediate appearance that is a combination of the two component beats)	No capture or fusion beats
ECG pattern	May be RBBB or LBBB	Usually RBBB
Concordance	Present (the QRS complexes retain the same axis throughout the chest leads)	Absent (some QRS complexes will be positive, others will be negative)
QRS waveform	May vary from beat to beat	Constant

AV, antrioventricular; LBBB, left bundle branch block; RBBB, right bundle branch block.

with aberrant conduction (or bundle branch block) (Fig. 12.3). This causes much confusion and concern amongst junior doctors and final-year students alike. It helps if you remember the following points:

- Both arrhythmias are potentially fatal so treat each with respect.
- The use of carotid sinus massage or adenosine may briefly block the atrioventricular node and, therefore, slow the ventricular response in supraventricular tachycardia (it will have no effect on VT).
- Never use verapamil or lidocaine (lignocaine) to slow the ventricular response in this situation: the negative inotropic effect of this drug could have disastrous effects if the rhythm is, in fact, VT, causing rapid development of cardiac failure.

Management

VT is very dangerous and if allowed to continue will result in cardiac failure or even death. Treatment must, therefore, be prompt and the nature of the treatment depends upon the clinical scenario:

- Patient conscious with VT and no haemodynamic compromise – treatment should be with drugs (these are discussed on p. 103).
- Patient conscious with VT, but haemodynamic compromise – triggered (synchronized) direct current (DC) cardioversion under general anaesthetic (fast bleep the anaesthetist).
- Patient unconscious with ongoing VT and no cardiac output ('pulseless VT') – praecordial

thump followed by triggered (synchronized) DC cardioversion as per cardiac arrest protocol (see Resuscitation Council guidelines Ch. 13).

It is vital to correct hypokalaemia promptly for all patients who have ventricular arrhythmias – potassium can be given orally or in a very dilute form via a peripheral vein. In the emergency situation larger doses of potassium can be given via a central line with careful monitoring of cardiac rhythm and serum potassium levels. Warning: intravenous potassium can cause ventricular fibrillation.

Electrophysiological studies

These studies involve inserting multiple electrodes into the heart via the great veins and positioning them at various intracardiac sites. Electrical activity can then be recorded from the atria, ventricles, bundle of His and so on to provide information on the type of conduction defect or rhythm disturbance. These studies are used mostly:

- to elucidate the mechanism of tachyarrhythmias
- therapeutically to terminate a tachyarrhythmia by overdrive pacing or shock

- therapeutically to ablate an area of myocardium thought to be propagating a recurrent tachyarrhythmia
- diagnostically to evaluate the risk of sudden cardiac death in patients who have possible ventricular tachyarrhythmias
- diagnostically to determine conduction defects in patients who have recurrent syncope.

Increasingly nowadays, patients who have survived a cardiac arrest will be treated with an implantable cardioverter defibrillator (ICD) without an electrophysiological study beforehand (see p. 105).

VENTRICULAR FIBRILLATION

Ventricular fibrillation (VF) is irregular rapid ventricular depolarization (Fig. 12.4). There is no organized contraction of the ventricle; therefore the patient has no pulse. This arrhythmia rapidly causes loss of consciousness and cardiorespiratory arrest.

Clinical features

The most common cause of VF is acute MI. However, it is also seen at the end-stage of many disease processes and signifies the presence of severe myocardial damage (this is sometimes referred to as secondary VF and usually results in death despite resuscitation attempts). It may be precipitated by:

- a ventricular ectopic beat
- ventricular tachycardia
- torsades de pointes.

Management

VF must be treated promptly with a praecordial thump and if this is unsuccessful with simple (non-synchronized) DC cardioversion (the resuscitation protocol is discussed in Ch. 13).

For secondary prevention an ICD is indicated (see p. 105).

Torsades de pointes

This rhythm is usually self-terminating, but can occasionally lead to VF and death. It is an irregular rapid rhythm with a characteristic twisting axis seen on the ECG (Fig. 12.5). In between episodes the ECG shows a long QT interval.

The QT interval corresponds to the time from depolarization to repolarization (beginning of the Q wave to end of T wave, i.e. action potential duration; see *Crash course: cardiovascular system*) and varies according to the heart rate. Therefore, a long QT interval is approximated by a corrected QT interval (QTc) of greater than 0.44 s. QTc = QT/square root of RR interval.

Clinical features

The patient usually feels faint or loses consciousness as the result of a drop in cardiac output. Attacks

Fig. 12.4 Ventricular fibrillation (VF) can have a coarse or a fine pattern.

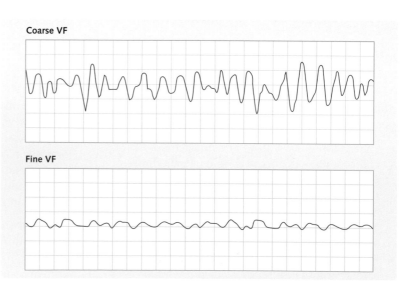

Coarse VF

Fine VF

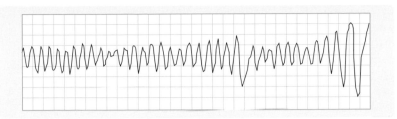

Fig. 12.5 Torsades de pointes. Note the irregular rhythm and twisting axis.

are much more likely to occur during periods of adrenergic stimulation (e.g. fear). There are many possible causes, all of which cause a prolonged QT interval (Fig. 12.6).

Management

Treatment of torsades de pointes differs from that of the other ventricular arrhythmias and is as follows:

Identify and treat any precipitating factors (stop offending drugs, correct electrolyte imbalance).

Atrial or ventricular pacing to maintain a heart rate of no less than 90 beats/min to prevent lengthening of the QT interval – intravenous isoprenaline may also be used to reduce the QT interval.

In congenital long QT syndromes high-dose β-blockers (β-adrenoceptor antagonists) or left stellectomy may be used and there is increasing use of permanent pacemakers and cardioverter defibrillators.

Do not use antiarrhythmic drugs.

DRUGS USED TO TREAT VENTRICULAR TACHYCARDIA AND FIBRILLATION

In the acute situation, if the patient is unconscious or has no cardiac output, a praecordial thump followed by DC cardioversion is used initially at 200 J. If the arrhythmia persists further resuscitation is carried out according to the set protocol. This is discussed in Chapter 13.

The drugs used to treat ventricular tachyarrhythmias other than torsades de pointes fall into two main classes:

1. Class I
2. Class III.

In the acutely ill patient who has VT or VF, antiarrhythmic agents may be given after sinus rhythm has been established by DC cardioversion (Fig. 12.7) in an effort to stabilize the myocardium. Amiodarone or β-blockers are commonly used, but

Fig. 12.6 Causes of a long QT interval

Cause	Examples
Congenital	Jervell and Lange–Nielsen syndrome (autosomal recessive and sensorineural deafness) Romano–Ward syndrome (autosomal dominant, no deafness)
Drugs	Class IA (e.g. quinidine, procainamide) Class III (e.g. amiodarone, sotalol) Tricyclic antidepressants (e.g. amitriptyline) Phenothiazines (e.g. chlorpromazine) Terfenadine
Electrolyte abnormalities	Hypokalaemia Hypomagnesaemia Hypocalcaemia
Others	Acute myocardial infarction Central nervous system disease Mitral valve prolapse Organophosphate insecticides

Fig. 12.7 Main features of common antiarrhythmic drugs classed using Vaughan Williams classification

Class of agent	Class I	Class II	Class III	Class IV	Digoxin
Examples	IA – quinidine, procainamide, disopyramide; IB – lidocaine (lignocaine) mexiletine, tocainide; IC – flecainide, propafenone	β-blockers (e.g. atenolol, bisoprolol, metoprolol); sotalol also has some class III activity	Amiodarone, sotalol, bretylium	Calcium channel blockers (e.g. diltiazem, verapamil)	Not classified by the Vaughan Williams system
Mode of action	Variable action on the His–Purkinje system	Increase AV node refractory period	Increase both AV node and His–Purkinje refractory period	Increase AV node refractory period	Slows AV conduction; increases AV node refractory period; positively inotropic
Adverse effects	Quinidine – nausea, diarrhoea; procainamide – development of antinuclear antibodies and SLE; flecainide – higher incidence of proarrhythmic effects than other class I drugs; all may lengthen QT and cause torsades; all are negatively inotropic	Negatively inotropic, may induce bronchospasm, exacerbation of peripheral vascular disease	Amiodarone – pulmonary fibrosis, hypo-/ hyperthyroidism, hepatic toxicity, cutaneous photosensitivity; corneal microdeposits (reversible), peripheral neuropathy; sotalol – as for other β-blockers; both may lengthen QT and cause torsades	Verapamil and diltiazem – complete AV block, negatively inotropic	Nausea, vomiting if blood levels too high, visual disturbances (xanthopsia), complete heart block positively inotropic

AV, atrioventricular; SLE, systemic lupus erythematosus

alternative agents include flecainide and lidocaine (lignocaine). Amiodarone is a good choice for the patient who has cardiac failure, because it has little negative inotropic effect. If given intravenously, amiodarone must be given centrally because it is extremely damaging to peripheral veins:

- Amiodarone has a very long half-life (25 days) and oral loading takes at least 1 month. Intravenous loading is faster.
- In a patient who has no contraindication for β-blockers, sotalol is a good long-term agent because it has none of the long-term side effects of amiodarone.
- Flecainide is an effective agent but is avoided in patients who have suspected ischaemic

heart disease because this may increase its proarrhythmic effects. For secondary prevention an ICD should be considered.

The Vaughan Williams classification of antiarrhythmic drugs allows agents to be grouped according to their mode of action on the myocardium and also makes selection of appropriate agents for the treatment of any given arrhythmia more straightforward.

Drug treatment alone for the secondary prevention of ventricular arrhythmia has been shown to be ineffective, although β-blockers should be used where possible in patients post MI or with heart failure, and drugs are a useful adjunct to reduce the frequency of arrhythmic events in conjunction with ICD therapy.

NON-PHARMACOLOGICAL TREATMENTS OF VENTRICULAR TACHYARRHYTHMIAS

Non-pharmacological treatments are used in patients who have recurrent VT or VF because:

- if successful, complete cure is achieved without the need for drugs
- localization of the arrhythmogenic focus is becoming possible in more cases due to increased understanding of the mechanisms of these arrhythmias.

The two methods commonly used are:

1. Radiofrequency ablation
2. Implantable cardioverter defibrillator (ICD).

Radiofrequency ablation

This involves localization of the proarrhythmic focus using intracardiac electrodes introduced via a central vein followed by the use of radiofrequency energy to cauterize the myocardium in that area. The successful result is the ablation of the focus, therefore rendering the patient cured and no longer needing antiarrhythmic agents. This technique is commonly used in patients who have Wolff–Parkinson–White syndrome (a supraventricular arrhythmia) who are young and have a discrete accessory pathway that can be localized easily. Ventricular arrhythmias can also sometimes be ablated.

Implantable cardioverter defibrillators

ICDs are now being increasingly used in the treatment of sustained or life-threatening ventricular arrhythmias, because they have been shown in some studies to prolong survival in such patients. These devices are slightly larger than a permanent pacemaker and are implanted in the same way (i.e. the box is situated superficial to the pectoralis major muscle on the patient's non-dominant side and the leads are positioned in the atrium and ventricle via the cephalic or subclavian vein). The device can sense VT and VF and can attempt to cardiovert the arrhythmia by pacing the ventricle or by delivering a DC shock.

The implantation and subsequent programming and monitoring of these devices should be performed in specialist centres. An ICD may be indicated for primary prevention (prophylaxis) as well as secondary prevention (previously documented episode).

Patients need counselling and advice before implantation of an ICD (in order to give fully informed consent) because the sensation when the ICD discharges a shock can be extremely unpleasant and comes without warning. This may result in marked psychological problems in some patients.

Further reading

Bardy G H, Lee K L, Mark D B et al 2005 Amiodarone or an implantable cardioverter-defibrillator for congestive heart failure. *N Engl J Med* **352**: 225–37

DiMarco J P 2003 Implantable cardioverter-defibrillators. *N Engl J Med* **349**: 1836–47

Edhouse J, Morris F March 2002 ABC of clinical electrocardiography: Broad complex tachycardia. *Part I, BMJ* **324**: 719–22, Part II, *BMJ* **324**: 776–9

Moss AJ, Zareba W, Hall WJ et al 2002 Prophylactic implantation of a defibrillator in patients with myocardial infarction and reduced ejection fraction. *N Engl J Med* **346**: 877–83

National Institute for Clinical Excellence 2000 Guidance on the use of implantable cardioverter defibrillators for arrhythmias. National Institute for Clinical Excellence, London

Fig. 13.1 Algorithm for adult basic life support.

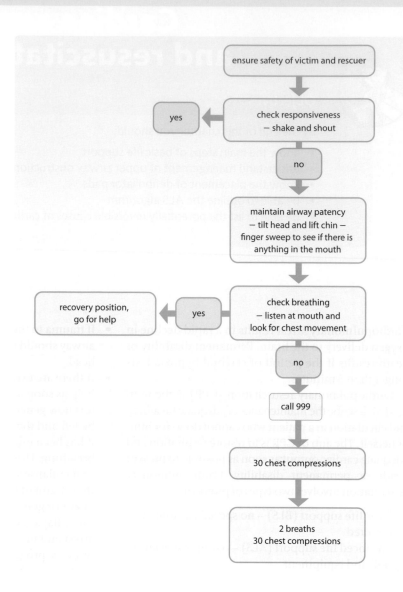

- The operator should be vertically above the victim's chest and the arms should be kept straight. The rate of compressions should be 100/min. After each compression the pressure should be released and the chest wall allowed to rise back up.

Principle of chest compressions

The current theory suggests that chest compression increases intrathoracic pressure and it is this that propels blood out of the thorax. The veins collapse, but the arteries remain patent and flow is, therefore, in a forward direction. The function and features of the recovery position are shown in Fig. 13.2.

The final examinations are likely to test BLS techniques, so practise these until you are competent. Inability to perform BLS satisfactorily in finals almost always results in a fail.

Management of upper airway obstruction by foreign material

The management of choking in a conscious victim, although not strictly BLS, is extremely important because it is a common occurrence both in the community and in the hospital where aspiration of stomach contents or blood may occur (Fig. 13.3).

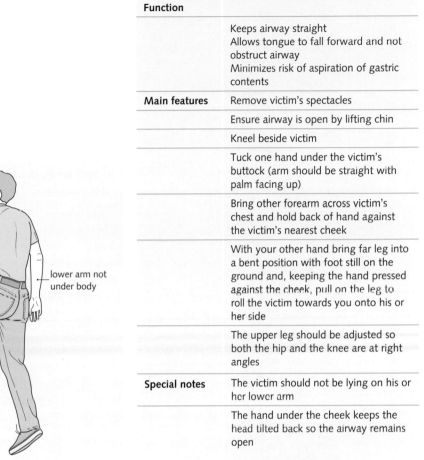

Fig. 13.2B Function and features of the recovery position

Function	
	Keeps airway straight Allows tongue to fall forward and not obstruct airway Minimizes risk of aspiration of gastric contents
Main features	Remove victim's spectacles
	Ensure airway is open by lifting chin
	Kneel beside victim
	Tuck one hand under the victim's buttock (arm should be straight with palm facing up)
	Bring other forearm across victim's chest and hold back of hand against the victim's nearest cheek
	With your other hand bring far leg into a bent position with foot still on the ground and, keeping the hand pressed against the cheek, pull on the leg to roll the victim towards you onto his or her side
	The upper leg should be adjusted so both the hip and the knee are at right angles
Special notes	The victim should not be lying on his or her lower arm
	The hand under the cheek keeps the head tilted back so the airway remains open

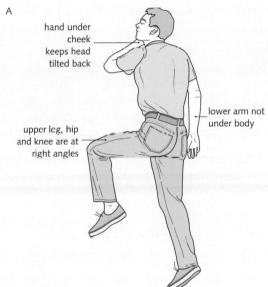

Fig. 13.2 (A) The recovery position viewed from above.

Points to note in the management of choking:

- If the patient becomes cyanosed then immediate positive action is needed with administration of oxygen and back blows followed by the Heimlich manoeuvre.
- Back blows are performed during expiration with the patient either standing or sitting, and with the head bent down below the level of the chest.
- Heimlich manoeuvre – this may be performed with the patient standing, sitting or lying down. Sharp upward pressure is applied in the midline just beneath the diaphragm with the operator behind the patient. This procedure can result in damage to abdominal viscera and should not be attempted in small children or pregnant women.

ADVANCED LIFE SUPPORT

The ALS method of resuscitation requires specialist training and equipment, and has recently been reviewed and modified. The 2005 Resuscitation Council (UK) guidelines use a universal algorithm that is dependent upon the presence or absence of a shockable or non-shockable rhythm (Fig. 13.4).

Make sure you have seen all of the pieces of equipment used for ALS.

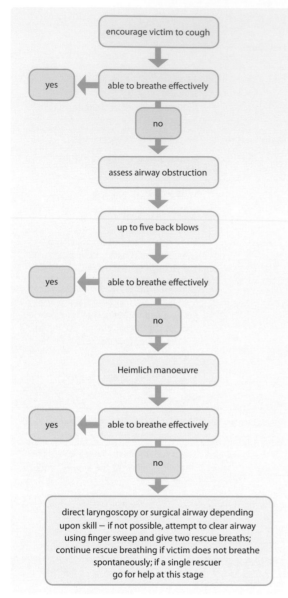

Fig. 13.3 Algorithm for the management of choking.

Following the shock, it is no longer advised to stop and check the rhythm. This is done at the end of the cycle of CPR. Adrenaline (10 ml of 1:10 000 i.v.) is given every 4 min (i.e. every two cycles) and atropine is only given in the event of a 'non-shockable' rhythm, such as PEA or asystole.

Airway ventilation and protection

During these cycles of CPR:

- adequate ventilation must be established
- the airway must be protected by an operator (preferably an anaesthetist) who remains at the patient's head.

The optimal method of protecting the airway is by insertion of a cuffed endotracheal tube. This device minimizes the risk of aspiration of the gastric contents and allows effective ventilation to be carried out. Endotracheal intubation can be a hazardous procedure and a laryngeal mask airway is an alternative.

Intravenous access must also be established either via a large peripheral vein or preferably via a central vein.

Placing the defibrillator paddles

Placement of the defibrillator paddles is important because only a small proportion of the energy reaches the myocardium during transthoracic defibrillation and every effort should be made to maximize this:

- The right paddle should be placed below the clavicle in the mid-clavicular line.
- The left paddle should be placed on the lower rib cage on the anterior axillary line.

Points to note about advanced life support

Protocol

The new protocol for ALS (see Further reading) consists of 2-min cycles of CPR (30 compression:2 breaths) irrespective of the initial rhythm. However, if the rhythm shows ventricular fibrillation (VF) or ventricular tachycardia (VT) (i.e. a 'shockable' rhythm) then the CPR is preceded by 1 shock.

Regardless of the setting, it is crucial that basic life support is commenced immediately and, once a cardiac monitor is available, that defibrillation of VT/VF is administered immediately. It is these two factors that affect the eventual outcome of resuscitation.

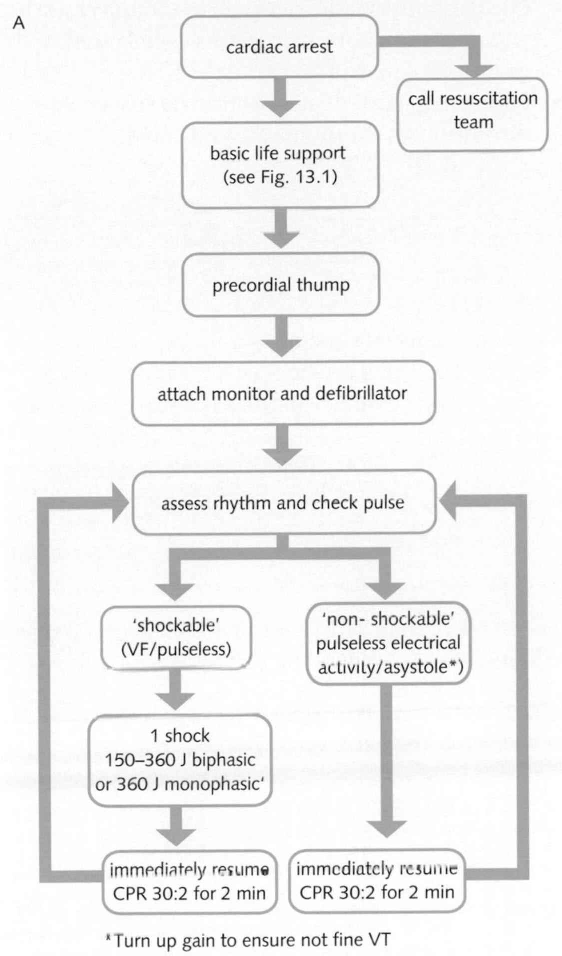

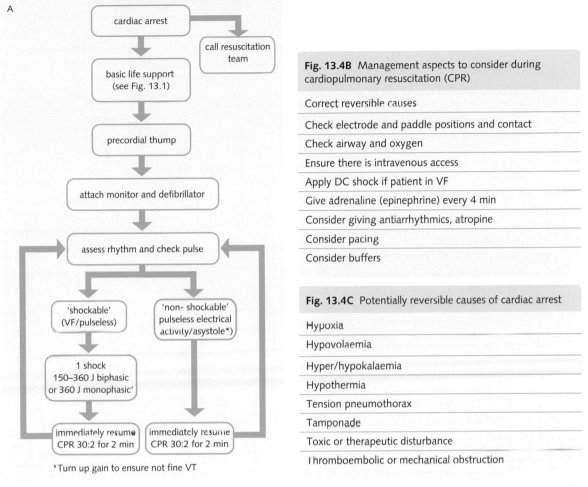

Fig. 13.4B Management aspects to consider during cardiopulmonary resuscitation (CPR)
Correct reversible causes
Check electrode and paddle positions and contact
Check airway and oxygen
Ensure there is intravenous access
Apply DC shock if patient in VF
Give adrenaline (epinephrine) every 4 min
Consider giving antiarrhythmics, atropine
Consider pacing
Consider buffers

Fig. 13.4C Potentially reversible causes of cardiac arrest
Hypoxia
Hypovolaemia
Hyper/hypokalaemia
Hypothermia
Tension pneumothorax
Tamponade
Toxic or therapeutic disturbance
Thromboembolic or mechanical obstruction

Fig. 13.4 (A) Algorithm for advanced life support. (B) Management aspects to consider during cardiopulmonary resuscitation (CPR). (C) Potentially reversible cause of cardiac arrest. VF, ventricular fibrillation; VT, ventricular tachycardia.

The ventricular tachycardia/fibrillation arm of the advanced life support algorithm

In the event of in-hospital cardiac arrest or out-of-hospital arrest witnessed by a healthcare professional, then if the rhythm shows VF or VT (so-called 'shockable' rhythms), one DC shock should be administered. The energy should be 360 J for a monophasic defibrillator, or 150–200 J for a biphasic defibrillator. Following this shock, CPR should be continued immediately. Pulse and rhythm are then assessed after one cycle of 2 min CPR. The algorithm then restarts with one further shock if indicated, or continuation of CPR for a further 2 min. Adrenaline is given every 4 min:

- If the arrhythmia persists, antiarrhythmics such as amiodarone may be used.

The non-VT/VF arm of the ALS algorithm

This arm includes asystole, pulseless electrical activity (previously termed electromechanical dissociation) and profound bradyarrhythmias. Prognosis for patients in this arm is much poorer than in the VF/VT arm. Defibrillation is not required unless VT/VF supervenes and 2-min cycles of CPR are given. During this period, possible underlying causes must be excluded or treated:

- Asystole is treated initially with i.v. atropine at a maximum total dose of 3 mg and i.v. adrenaline 1 mg. During subsequent cycles of CPR adrenaline may be repeated, but not the atropine.

- Bradyarrhythmias are treated initially with atropine in the same way. Patients who have bradyarrhythmia may benefit from insertion of a temporary pacing wire.

Pulseless electrical activity (PEA) occurs when there is a regular rhythm on the monitor (that is not VT), but no cardiac output arising from it. Underlying causes must be sought because these may be easily treated. The following are possible underlying causes of EMD:

- Hypovolaemia – rapid administration of i.v. fluids is required.
- Electrolyte imbalance (e.g. hypokalaemia, hypocalcaemia) – check ABG.
- Tension pneumothorax – suspect in trauma cases or after insertion of central line; also seen spontaneously in fit young men. Look for absence of chest movements and breath sounds on one side. Treat with cannula into the pleural space at the second intercostal space in mid-clavicular line followed by insertion of chest drain.

- Cardiac tamponade – suspect in trauma cases and post-thoracotomy patients. Need rapid insertion of pericardial drain.
- Pulmonary embolism – if strongly suspected thrombolysis should be administered.

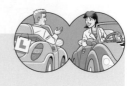

It is helpful in the event of a cardiac arrest for an experienced member of the team to discuss the course of events early on with the patient's relatives or next of kin if possible. Discussing the situation at an early stage can facilitate breaking bad news if the resuscitation attempt is unsuccessful.

Further reading

Resuscitation Council (UK) 2005 Adult Advanced Life Support Resuscitation Guidelines http://www.resus.org.uk/pages/mediMain.htm

Resuscitation Council (UK) http://www.resus.org.uk/

Bradyarrhythmias

Objectives

By the end of this chapter you should:

- know the pathological causes of sinus bradycardia
- understand the difference between Mobitz I and Mobitz II heart block and how they are managed
- be able to describe the management of complete heart block
- be able to recognize the ECG appearance of left bundle branch block
- be aware of different types of pacemakers.

DEFINITION OF BRADYARRHYTHMIAS

The bradyarrhythmias (Fig. 14.1) are slow rhythms.

SINUS BRADYCARDIA

Sinus bardycardia occurs when the resting heart rate is less than 60 beats/min; this can be physiological (e.g. during sleep) and is also seen in young athletes. Pathological causes include:

- sinus node disease (especially in the elderly)
- raised intracranial pressure
- severe hypoxia
- hypothyroidism (myxoedema)
- hypothermia
- tumours (cervical, mediastinal)
- sepsis
- drugs (β-blockers, calcium channel blockers and other antiarrhythmic agents)
- ischaemic heart disease affecting the SA node (in 60% of patients the SA node is supplied by the right coronary artery).

Patients are usually asymptomatic and no treatment is required. Occasionally, however, syncope, hypotension or dyspnoea may occur. In these circumstances, treatment with i.v. atropine or isoprenaline, or insertion of a temporary pacing wire might be required to speed up the heart rate until the underlying condition is treated.

Sinus node disease

The sinoatrial (SA) node is the natural cardiac pacemaker. It is a crescent-shaped structure approximately 1 mm × 3 mm in size. The SA node is located just below the epicardial surface at the junction of the right atrium and the superior vena cava.

The rate at which the SA node generates impulses is determined by both vagal and sympathetic tone. The impulses are conducted via the atrial myocardium to the atrioventricular (AV) node.

Disease of the SA node may be due to:

- ischaemia and infarction
- degeneration and fibrosis
- excessive vagal stimulation
- myocarditis.

This can result in pauses between consecutive P waves (>2 s). There are degrees of SA node conduction abnormality:

- Sinoatrial exit block – an expected P wave is absent, but the following one occurs at the expected time (i.e. the pauses are exact multiples of the basic PP interval).
- Sinus pause or sinus arrest (Fig. 14.2) – the interval between the P waves is longer than 2 s and is not a multiple of the basic PP interval.

Tachy-brady syndrome (sick sinus syndrome)

This is a combination of sinus node disease and abnormal tachyarrhythmias. Ischaemia is a common

Fig. 14.1 Bradyarrhythmias listed in ascending order of electrical dysfunction

Bradyarrhythmia	Features
Sinus bradycardia	Heart rate <60 beats/min during the day
Sinoatrial node disease and sick sinus syndrome	Prolonged PP interval, may be associated with tachyarrhythmias and, intermittently, with tachy-brady syndrome
First-degree heart block Second-degree heart block – Mobitz type I	PR interval >0.20 s Wenckebach phenomenon – progressive prolongation of PR interval with eventual dropped beat
Second-degree heart block – Mobitz type II	Dropped beats, no prolongation of PR interval
Second-degree heart block – 2:1 heart block/3:1 heart block	Every second or third beat conducted, the rest are not
Complete heart block, third degree heart block	Complete AV dissociation
Asystole	No beats conducted, no ventricular activity
Ventricular standstill P wave aystole	Visible P waves but no QRS complex

AV, atrioventricular.

Fig. 14.2 Sinus pause or arrest. Note the interval of more than 2 s between P waves.

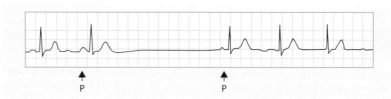

P   P

Management

Patients who have symptomatic sinus pauses or evidence of recurrent sinus pauses require permanent pacing with a dual-chamber pacemaker (assuming rate-slowing drugs have been discontinued). Single chamber (ventricular) pacemakers are usually reserved only for patients who have atrial fibrillation.

Antiarrhythmic drugs may also be needed if the patient has sick sinus syndrome. Pacemaker insertion should be considered before commencing these because they will make the SA node conduction defect worse.

ATRIOVENTRICULAR BLOCK

The AV node is a complex structure that lies in the right atrial wall on the septal surface between the ostium of the coronary sinus and the septal leaflet of the tricuspid valve. In 90% of patients the AV node is supplied by the right coronary artery. The rest are supplied via the circumflex coronary artery.

The AV node acts as a physiological gearbox conducting impulses from the atria to the ventricular conductive tissue.

First-degree atrioventricular block

In this conduction disturbance (Fig. 14.3), conduction time through the AV node is prolonged, but all impulses are conducted. The PR interval is longer than 0.20 s.

This condition does not require treatment in a healthy patient, but should be watched because it can herald greater degrees of block (this occurs in approximately 40% of cases). This is particularly important in patients who have evidence of other conducting tissue disease, e.g. bundle branch block.

cause for this syndrome, which occurs in the elderly.

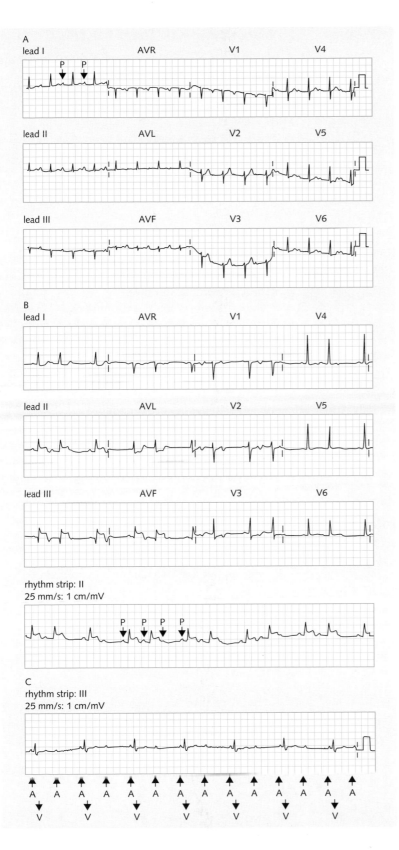

115

Second-degree atrioventricular block

In this type of block some impulses are not conducted from the atria to the ventricles.

Mobitz type 1 heart block – Wenckebach phenomenon

Wenckebach phenomenon is characterized by progressive prolongation of the PR interval; eventually resulting in a non-conducted P wave (dropped QRS complex). The cycle is then repeated. This is a common phenomenon and can occur in any cardiac tissue, including the SA node.

In a patient who has infective endocarditis serial ECGs are performed to observe the PR interval. Prolongation of this can occur secondary to the formation of a paravalvular abscess (the conducting tissue is in close proximity to the valve ring) and this usually heralds rapid development of complete heart block and valve dehiscence. In these patients progressive prolongation of the PR interval therefore requires an urgent ECG and temporary pacing wire.

Wenckebach phenomenon can occur in athletes and children, and is due to high vagal tone. It is usually benign and is not usually an indication for pacing.

When it occurs after an inferior myocardial infarction (MI), pacing is not usually required unless the patient is symptomatic. In anterior MI any newly developed heart block suggests massive septal necrosis and temporary pacing is required.

Mobitz type II heart block

The PR interval remains constant and P waves are dropped intermittently. This type of heart block carries a risk of progressing to complete heart block and requires insertion of a pacemaker.

2:1 or 3:1 heart block

This represents a more advanced degree of block and requires pacing because there is a high risk of complete heart block.

Third-degree or complete heart block

Complete heart block (Fig. 14.4) results in dissociation of the atria from the ventricles.

The ECG shows the P waves and the QRS waves are independent from each other. The P and QRS complexes are regular, but bear no temporal relationship to one another. There is a ventricular 'escape' rhythm, which usually gives rise to wide QRS complexes.

On examination there might be some classic features:

- The first heart sound has a variable intensity.
- There are intermittent cannon waves in the jugular venous pulse. These correspond to a large a wave caused by the right atrial contraction against a closed tricuspid valve.

Management depends upon the underlying cause:

- After an inferior MI a temporary pacemaker should be inserted in the event of haemodynamic compromise. A significant proportion of these cases revert back to normal conduction within a few weeks and a permanent pacemaker is often not needed. If the heart block is due to drugs

Fig. 14.4 Complete heart block. Atrial P waves (A) and ventricular QRS (V) complexes are completely dissociated.

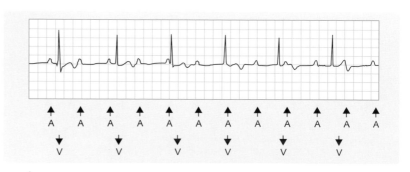

(e.g. β-blockers) it may resolve once these are withdrawn.

- After an anterior MI or in any other situation a permanent pacemaker will be required and should be inserted immediately (unless the patient is unstable in which case a temporary wire is inserted first followed by a permanent system some days later).

Bradyarrhythmias do not usually compromise cardiac output if the rate is over 50/min and the ventricles have normal function.

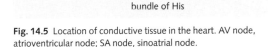

Fig. 14.5 Location of conductive tissue in the heart. AV node, atrioventricular node; SA node, sinoatrial node.

BUNDLE BRANCH BLOCK

Bundle branch block is an interventricular conduction disturbance. The bundle of His arises from the AV node and at the level of the top of the muscular interventricular septum it divides into the left and right bundle branches (Fig. 14.5), which supply the left and right ventricles, respectively. The left bundle divides again into anterior and posterior divisions.

Damage to one or more of these bundles due to ischaemia or infarction (or any other condition disturbing electrical conduction; see SA node disease,

above) results in a characteristic ECG picture as the pattern of depolarization of the ventricles is altered.

In either complete left or complete right bundle branch block the QRS complex is widened to greater than 0.12 s.

Left bundle branch block

In the normal situation the septum is depolarized from left to right. If the left bundle is blocked the septum is depolarized from right to left and the right ventricle depolarized before the left. This results in the classic M-shaped complex in lead V6 (Fig. 14.6).

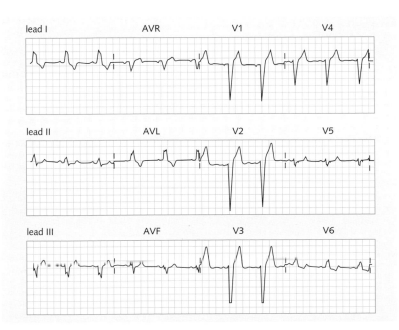

Fig. 14.6 Complete left bundle branch block. This is characterized by widening of the QRS complex. The R wave is positive in I (to the left) and negative in V1 (posterior) (i.e. the delayed depolarization is to the left ventricle). Note the widened complexes and the M-shaped complexes in V6.

Remember that V6 is on the left side of the chest and that a positive deflection occurs when current flows towards the lead. The initial upstroke is due to septal depolarization from right to left and, therefore, towards lead V6. Depolarization of the right ventricle occurs next, which is in a centre to right direction and, therefore, causes a negative deflection. Finally, the left ventricle is depolarized, which is from right to left, causing the final upstroke.

It is possible to see isolated block of the left anterior or left posterior fascicles of the left bundle branch on the ECG. Left anterior hemiblock causes a left axis deviation on the ECG and left posterior hemiblock causes right axis deviation.

Right bundle branch block

This results in the classic RSR pattern in leads V1 and V2 (Fig. 14.7), which lie to the right of the left ventricle. The septum is depolarized from left to right as normal (resulting in an upstroke in V1), but as there is no conduction down the right bundle the left ventricle depolarizes first, which causes a current to the left resulting in a negative stroke in V1. Finally, the delayed right ventricular depolarization of the right ventricle occurs, causing another upstroke in V1.

> Bundle branch block may progress to complete heart block; intermittent heart block should be suspected in patients who present with syncope and bundle branch block.

INVESTIGATION OF BRADYARRHYTHMIAS

Electrocardiography

This may show evidence of heart block. However, if the heart block is intermittent the ECG may be normal.

In a patient who has unexplained syncope it is important to exclude intermittent conduction disturbances using continuous ambulatory ECG monitoring. These devices can be used to record the ECG over at least 24 h continuously.

Blood tests

Liver function and thyroid function tests may reveal causes of sinus bradycardia.

Fig. 14.7 Right bundle branch block. Note the wide QRS. The late part of the QRS in time is negative in I (i.e. to the right) and positive in V1 (i.e. anterior). The delayed depolarization is to the right ventricle. Note the widened QRS complexes and the RSR pattern in V1 and V2.

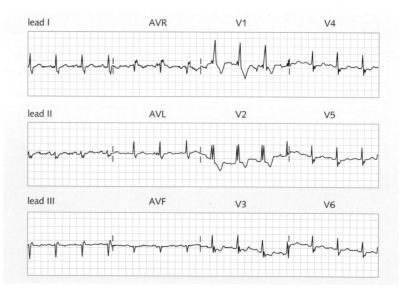

Chest radiography

This may reveal cardiomegaly in patients who have ischaemic cardiomyopathy or myocarditis. Pulmonary oedema may be a result of the bradycardia.

Echocardiography

This may reveal regional wall hypokinesia due to areas of ischaemia or infarction. This is especially relevant if it involves the septum.

PACEMAKERS

Indications for a permanent pacemaker

A pacemaker is used to deliver electrical stimuli via leads in contact with the heart. The leads not only deliver energy, but are also able to sense spontaneous electrical activity from the heart. The aim of inserting a pacemaker is to mimic as closely as possible the normal electrical activity of the heart in a patient who has a potentially life-threatening conduction disturbance. The indications for a permanent pacemaker are listed in Fig. 14.8.

Indications for temporary pacing

The following indications for temporary pacing are appropriate:

- All of the above (see Fig. 14.8) if there is no facility for permanent pacing immediately available
- Drug-induced symptomatic bradyarrhythmias – a temporary wire is used until the effect of the drug has worn off, for example after a trial or overdose of a β-blocker (β-adrenoceptor antagonist)
- Heart block after inferior MI if there is haemodynamic compromise.

Pacemaker insertion

Both temporary and permanent pacemakers are inserted via a venous route by introducing first a sheath and then a pacing wire into one of the great veins.

Permanent pacemakers are most often inserted into the cephalic or subclavian veins. In an emergency situation a temporary wire may be inserted into the internal jugular, subclavian or femoral vein (using the Seldinger technique).

In the case of the temporary pacemaker, the pacemaker box sits externally. In the case of the permanent pacemaker it is buried under the fat and subcutaneous tissue overlying one of the pectoralis major muscles (usually on the patient's non-dominant side).

Complications of pacemaker insertion

The following are recognized complications of pacemaker insertion:

Fig. 14.8 Indications for a permanent pacemaker

- Complete AV block – should be permanently paced whether symptomatic or not unless following inferior MI (may recover)
- Mobitz type II block and 2:1 and 3:1 block with symptoms
- Symptomatic bifascicular BBB (i.e. RBBB and left anterior or posterior hemiblock)
- Trifascicular block, if symptomatic (i.e. first-degree heart block, RBBB and left anterior or posterior hemiblock)
- Sinus node pauses ± tachycardia
- Symptomatic sinus bradycardia with no treatable cause
- After inferior MI with persistent complete heart block or persistent Mobitz type II block after trial with temporary pacing wire
- After anterior MI with persistent complete heart block or persistent Mobitz type II block: trial with temporary pacing is unnecessary as conduction very rarely recovers
- Symptomatic bradyarrhythmia following drug treatment of a serious tachyarrhythmia; continue the antiarrhythmic drug and combine with a permanent pacemaker

MI, myocardial infarction; RBBB, right bundle branch block.

Fig. 14.9 Classification of pacemakers.

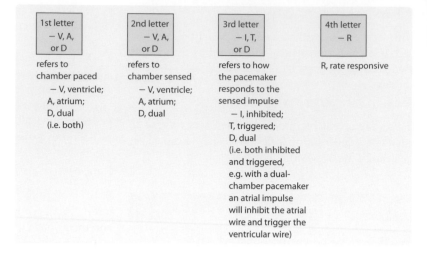

1st letter — V, A, or D	2nd letter — V, A, or D	3rd letter — I, T, or D	4th letter — R
refers to chamber paced — V, ventricle; A, atrium; D, dual (i.e. both)	refers to chamber sensed — V, ventricle; A, atrium; D, dual	refers to how the pacemaker responds to the sensed impulse — I, inhibited; T, triggered; D, dual (i.e. both inhibited and triggered, e.g. with a dual-chamber pacemaker an atrial impulse will inhibit the atrial wire and trigger the ventricular wire)	R, rate responsive

- Complications of wire insertion such as pneumothorax, haemorrhage, brachial plexus injury (during subclavian vein puncture), arrhythmias as the wire is manipulated inside the heart and infection (may progress to infective endocarditis).
- Complications of permanent pacemaker box positioning (e.g. haematoma formation, infection and erosion of the box through the skin).
- Difficulties with the wire, such as wire displacement and loss of ability to pace or sense (need to reposition wire), fracture of the wire insulation (usually due to tight sutures or friction against the clavicle – need to replace wire) and perforation of the myocardium (uncommon unless after MI when the myocardium is friable – need to reposition wire).

Types of pacemaker

Pacemakers are classified according to a four-letter code (Fig. 14.9).

Ventricular pacemakers stimulate ventricular contraction only and patients who have these, have no atrial contribution to the cardiac output. The atrial contribution can, however, be very important (up to 25% of total cardiac output). It is generally accepted now that a dual-chamber pacemaker should be fitted in patients in whom the atrium can be paced and sensed.

Patients who have chronic atrial fibrillation cannot have an atrial wire because the constant random electrical activity cannot be appropriately sensed.

Pacemaker syndrome

Permanent single-chamber right ventricular pacing in a patient who has intact atrial function can lead to atrial activation by retrograde conduction from the ventricle – so-called pacemaker syndrome. There is a cannon wave with every beat, pulmonary arterial pressure rises and cardiac output is impaired. This is managed by replacing the pacemaker with a dual-chamber device.

Patients must be informed of the need to notify the DVLA following pacemaker insertion as they will not be allowed to drive until after a pacemaker check is carried out at follow-up.

Further reading

ACC/AHA/NASPE Committee Members, and Task Force Members October 2002 ACC/AHA/NASPE 2002 Guideline update for implantation of cardiac pacemakers and antiarrhythmia devices. *Circulation* **106**: 2145–61

Da Costa D, Brady W J, Edhouse J March 2002 ABC of clinical electrocardiography: bradycardias and atrioventricular conduction block. *BMJ* **324**: 535–8

Mangrum J M, DiMarco J P March 2000 The evaluation and management of bradycardia. *N Engl J Med* **342**: 703–9

Cardiac failure

Objectives

By the end of this chapter you should:

- be able to list the main causes of heart failure and understand the mechanisms by which it develops
- be able to recognize the main clinical signs of left-ventricular and right-ventricular failure
- know the management steps of acute pulmonary oedema
- be able to list the drugs used in the treatment of chronic heart failure.

DEFINITION OF CARDIAC FAILURE

Cardiac failure is the inability of the heart to perfuse metabolizing tissues adequately. The most common cause of this is myocardial failure, which can be caused by a wide variety of disease states.

Myocardial failure can affect the left and right ventricles individually or both together. If left untreated, left-ventricular failure (LVF) will lead to right-ventricular failure (RVF) due to high right-ventricular pressure load. Very occasionally there is no abnormality of myocardial function, but cardiac failure occurs. This is due to a sudden excessive high demand on the heart (Fig. 15.1) or acute pressure load.

The remainder of this chapter discusses myocardial failure.

PATHOPHYSIOLOGY OF CARDIAC FAILURE

Normal myocardial response to work

During exercise and other stresses there is an increased adrenergic stimulation of the myocardium and cardiac pacemaker tissue. This results in tachycardia and increased myocardial contractility.

An increase in venous return causes an increased end-diastolic volume of the left ventricle resulting in stretching of the myocytes. This stretch causes an increase in myocardial performance – as predicted by the Frank-Starling law (Fig. 15.2).

The terms 'preload' and 'afterload' are commonly used. Load is a force – in this case the force in the wall of the cardiac chambers. Preload = diastolic force. Afterload = systolic force. Preload and afterload always change together because of the LaPlace relationship (e.g. increasing venous return increases volume and, therefore, systolic wall force). Vasodilatation shifts blood from the heart and decreases diastolic and systolic wall force.

At the same time, vasodilatation in the exercising muscles reduces peripheral vascular resistance resulting in a marked increase in cardiac output with relatively little increase in systemic blood pressure.

The failing heart's response to work

The adrenergic system is already at an increased level of activity in cardiac failure in an attempt to boost cardiac output. During stress this stimulation increases, but cardiac reserve does not permit a significant increase in contractility. The result is tachycardia with its increased energy

Fig. 15.4A Consequences of left and right ventricular failure

	LV failure	RV failure
Symptoms	Dyspnoea secondary to pulmonary oedema and lactic acidosis	Dyspnoea secondary to poor pulmonary perfusion
	Fatigue due to poor cardiac output and lactic acidosis	Fatigue due to poor LV filling (and therefore poor cardiac output and lactic acidosis)
Signs	Hypotension, cold peripheries and renal impairment – all due to poor LV output	Hypotension and cold peripheries due to poor LV filling (and therefore poor LV output)
	LV third heart sound – heard best at the apex	RV third heart sound – very soft and best heard at the left lower sternal edge
	Bilateral basal crepitations	Elevated JVP
	Signs of CCF – severe chronic LV failure leads to fluid retention	Ascites, hepatic enlargement and peripheral oedema

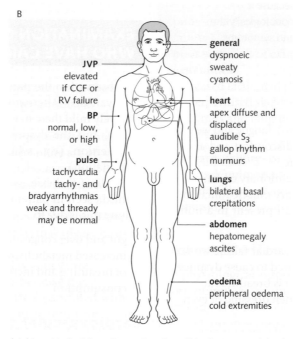

B

JVP
elevated
if CCF or
RV failure

BP
normal, low,
or high

pulse
tachycardia
tachy- and
bradyarrhythmias
weak and thready
may be normal

general
dyspnoeic
sweaty
cyanosis

heart
apex diffuse and
displaced
audible S₃
gallop rhythm
murmurs

lungs
bilateral basal
crepitations

abdomen
hepatomegaly
ascites

oedema
peripheral oedema
cold extremities

Fig. 15.4 (A) Consequences of left and right ventricular failure. One or the other will be dominant and the clinical picture varies accordingly. Often there are signs of both. CCF, congestive cardiac failure; JVP, jugular venous pressure; LV, left ventricular; RV, right ventricular. (B) Clinical findings in a patient who has heart failure. BP, blood pressure; CCF, congestive cardiac failure; RV, right ventricular.

If a raised JVP is non-pulsatile, consider superior vena caval obstruction.
A pulsatile raised JVP with no oedema means tricuspid regurgitation and, therefore, right heart failure. A pulsatile raised JVP with oedema is usually due to congestive cardiac failure, but right-heart failure is revealed if the JVP remains high after removal of the oedema with diuretics.

- carotid pulse – look for abnormal pulse character because it may reveal a possible aetiology for the cardiac failure (e.g. aortic stenosis or regurgitation)
- apex beat – may be displaced downward and laterally in a patient who has an enlarged left ventricle. A diffuse apex beat is a sign of severe left-ventricular dysfunction
- heart sounds – on auscultation there may be a third heart sound. Tachycardia combined with a third (or fourth heart sound) is referred to as a gallop rhythm

- murmurs – these may signify a possible cause of cardiac failure (e.g. aortic valve murmurs and mitral valve murmurs). Remember: mitral regurgitation can occur as a result of left-ventricular dilatation (which leads to stretching of the mitral valve ring) and will, therefore, be caused by cardiac failure, and not a cause of it, in some cases. This is called functional mitral regurgitation
- peripheral oedema – this may be elicited over the sacrum or over the ankle. Take care because oedema may be tender. The extent to which the oedema extends up the legs is an indication of the extent of the fluid overload.

Respiratory system

In addition to dyspnoea and possible cyanosis, the patient might have bilateral basal fine end-inspiratory crepitations extending from the bases upwards. This is classic of pulmonary oedema. There might also be pleural effusions and expiratory wheeze (secondary to cardiac asthma).

Dyspnoea secondary to pulmonary oedema is worse on lying flat and in severe cases the patient has to sit upright. In this situation it is reasonable not to ask the patient to sit at 45° and to conduct the examination in the upright position.

Gastrointestinal system

Patients with CCF or pure RVF might show signs of hepatomegaly and ascites.

Take care when palpating the liver or attempting to elicit the hepatojugular reflex, because CCF can result in tender hepatomegaly.

INVESTIGATION OF CARDIAC FAILURE

Blood tests

Electrolytes and renal function

Hypokalaemia and hyponatraemia are common findings in patients who are on diuretic therapy. There may also be renal impairment due to hypoperfusion or diuretic therapy. Hyponatraemia may be found in patients who are not on diuretics due to sodium restriction and high circulating vasopressin levels (dilutional hyponatraemia).

Hyperkalaemia may be seen in patients who are being treated with potassium-sparing diuretics (e.g. amiloride or spironolactone), angiotensin-converting enzyme (ACE) inhibitors (e.g. ramipril or perindopril) or angiotensin II receptor blockers (ARBs), such as losartan or candesartan.

Full blood count

Chronic anaemia may lead to cardiac failure. There may be a leucocytosis secondary to infection, which may exacerbate cardiac failure.

Liver function tests

Liver congestion may lead to impaired hepatic function, resulting in elevated hepatic enzymes and bilirubin.

Brain natriuretic peptide

Assays of BNP are increasingly used as a screening test for heart failure in the community, with serum levels elvated in heart failure. (See Neurohumoral factors, p. 123.)

Arterial blood gases

These show hypoxia, hypocapnoea and metabolic acidosis. Patients who are profoundly hypoxic might require artificial ventilation.

Electrocardiography

This may be normal or may show ischaemic or hypertensive changes. Look out for evidence of arrhythmias. If these are suspected, a 24-h ECG should be performed.

Chest radiography

There may be cardiomegaly indicating a dilated left ventricle. Pulmonary oedema may be seen with prominent pulmonary veins, upper lobe blood diversion and Kerley B lines (horizontal lines of fluid-filled fissures at the costophrenic angle).

Echocardiography

This is an essential test in heart failure; it is non-invasive and can be performed on and off the ward. It can help to determine:

- left and right ventricular dimensions and function
- abnormalities of regional wall motion caused by ischaemia
- any structural or functional abnormalities for all valves
- pressure differences across narrowed valves and also estimation of pulmonary artery pressure.
- intracardiac thrombus (although transoesophageal echocardiography is more sensitive for that purpose)
- Exclusion of intracardiac shunt.

Cardiac catheterization

It is important to evaluate underlying coronary artery disease as a cause of heart failure as coronary revascularization (where necessary) may improve the pumping ability of the heart. This is usually performed when heart failure symptoms have been stabilized with medical therapy, unless there is objective evidence of acute ischaemia.

MANAGEMENT OF CARDIAC FAILURE

The most common clinical presentation seen in the outpatients department and on the ward is the patient who has chronic LVF or CCF (heart failure with fluid retention).

Before discussing this, two clinical situations will be covered because they are both emergencies and make good viva questions to ask in finals. These are:

1. management of acute LVF
2. management of acute RVF.

Management of acute left ventricular failure

Acute LVF is a very common condition and is also a medical emergency. Rapid venodilatation is required to remove blood and fluid from the chest. It is, therefore, important that you know all the management steps in Fig. 15.5, including drugs and doses, before finals. If the patient is extremely unwell and may need endotracheal intubation, an anaesthetist should be called immediately.

This is a medical emergency that you will almost certainly encounter in your first year as an FI. You will be expected to administer all first-line treatment by yourself so it is important to know not only the drugs to use, but also all the doses and routes of administration. This tends to be a pass/fail question in vivas.

The patient in acute LVF has pulmonary oedema and is very breathless and distressed. He or she will be hypoxic and may cough up pink frothy sputum. Forward failure may be present leading to hypotension.

Your aim is to relieve the pulmonary oedema rapidly.

If the patient has cardiogenic shock and is very hypotensive, inotropic agents may be needed and you should call your registrar or senior house officer immediately because in this situation the blood pressure should be improved first.

Learn the management guide given in Fig. 15.5.

Management of acute right ventricular failure

Patients with an inferior or posterior myocardial infarction (MI) may present with predominantly RVF. This is not common, but it is important to recognize the signs and to know how to treat it.

Remember Starling's law of the heart, where the force of contraction is proportional to the stretch applied to the muscle. It is often possible to improve function by increasing heart volume (unless the ventricle is severely dysfunctional, in which case this makes no difference).

Treatment of acute RVF can be opposite to that of acute LVF. Fluid administration may be needed in RVF. In LVF the fluid needs to be removed.

Remember that, unlike LVF, isolated RVF is very rare and is more commonly found in association with LVF.

In the post-MI patient, dehydration, diuretic use and the use of nitrates are all common. All of these conspire to reduce heart volume.

Fig. 15.5 Management of acute left ventricular failure (LVF)

Management (in order)	Notes
1. Sit the patient up	To reduce venous return to the heart
2. Administer 100% oxygen via a facial mask	Improvement of arterial oxygen tension will reduce myocardial oxygen debt and improve myocardial function
3. Establish peripheral intravenous access and administer:	
IV diamorphine 2.5–5 mg	Diamorphine is a good anxiolytic and also a venodilator, so reducing load
IV metoclopramide 10 mg	Metoclopramide prevents vomiting secondary to diamorphine
IV furosemide (frusemide) 80–100 mg	Furosemide (frusemide) is a venodilator so its initial effect is to reduce load; it is also a powerful diuretic and will cause salt and water excretion, so reducing fluid retention
	By reducing load these drugs reduce the backpressure on the pulmonary circulation and hence relieve pulmonary oedema by allowing resorption of fluid back from the extracellular to the intracellular space
4. Insert a urinary catheter	The patient will have a diuresis and is too ill to use a bedpan; it is important to monitor fluid output to detect renal impairment early
5. Intravenous nitrates	Given as a continuous infusion; help by vasodilating both veins and arterioles and so reducing load; the dose is titrated to prevent hypotension (a common side-effect of nitrates)
6. CPAP	Very effective – it literally pushes fluid out of the alveoli back into the circulation; specialist equipment is required
	When the patient is stable, continue management as for chronic left ventricular failure

CPAP, continuous positive airway pressure; IV, intravenous.

If right-ventricular function is impaired a reduced heart volume has the effect of reducing function further, resulting in poor left-ventricular filling and hypotension. In fact, an impaired right ventricle requires greater than normal filling in order to maintain normal output.

Therefore, a patient who has an inferior MI and hypotension should be assessed carefully.

You must be aware that hypotension after inferior MI might be secondary to the combination of RVF and relative underfilling of the right ventricle, and that treatment is careful fluid challenge with central venous pressure monitoring.

Provided that there is no evidence of pulmonary oedema (suggesting the presence of significant left-ventricular impairment), the correct management is a gentle fluid challenge.

Management of chronic cardiac failure

The main agents used in the treatment of chronic cardiac failure are:

- ACE inhibitors (angiotensin II receptor blockers if patients are intolerant to ACE inhibitors)
- diuretics
- spironolactone
- β-blockers
- nitrates
- digoxin
- hydralazine.

A dilated heart means chronic rather than acute heart failure.

Angiotensin-converting enzyme inhibitors

The role of the renin-angiotensin system in cardiac failure is discussed on pp. 121–3. It is not difficult to see that inhibition of formation of angiotensin II could be beneficial by reducing systemic vasoconstriction and the sodium and water retention caused by aldosterone.

Angiotensin II increases efferent arteriolar tone and, therefore, increases glomerular filtration. Because ACE inhibitors remove this ability to regulate efferent arteriolar tone, the glomerular filtration rate declines and renal failure ensues in patients who have renal artery stenosis or any other condition in which renal blood flow is reduced (e.g. marked hypotension).

Examples of ACE inhibitors, grouped according to which part of the molecule binds the zinc moiety of ACE, are:

- captopril – has a sulfydryl group
- enalapril, lisinopril, ramipril – carboxyl group
- fosinopril – phosphinic acid.

The ACE inhibitors have been shown to reduce the mortality rate in patients who have heart failure. They are the first-line drugs for all patients who have heart failure, unless there is a specific contraindication (e.g. renal artery stenosis or profound hypotension).

Clinical use of angiotensin-converting enzyme inhibitors

ACE inhibitors are usually started at low doses because they can cause first-dose hypotension. Patients most likely to suffer from this are:

- the elderly
- patients who are on high doses of diuretics.

Once the dose has been established, renal function and electrolytes should be checked one week later to ensure no deterioration has taken place in renal function. Hyperkalaemia is another complication that is due to a reduction in aldosterone activity (aldosterone causes sodium absorption in exchange

for potassium in the distal convoluted tubule). Other side effects of ACE inhibitors are:

- cough – occurs in 5% patients on these agents. It is caused by inhibition of the metabolism of bradykinin (another function of ACE). Cough usually appears in the first few weeks of treatment. This is a side effect of all drugs in this class and treatment needs to be stopped in some cases
- loss of taste (or a metallic taste) may occur
- rashes and angioedema.

A multidisciplinary team approach is the key to the modern management of patients with heart failure. Nurse specialists in heart failure can optimize drug therapy and give education and lifestyle advice, and work in conjunction with physiotherapists, dietitians, pharmacists and physicians.

Once the drug has been introduced the dose should be increased to the recommended dose if possible (e.g. ramipril 10 mg daily or perindopril 8 mg daily).

Angiotensin II receptor blockers

There are two types of angiotensin II receptor: AT1 and AT2. Losartan is a selective AT1 blocker and was the first of these drugs to be established for use as an antihypertensive. Candesartan has been shown to benefit patients with heart failure; however, other agents are emerging and are being evaluated for similar benefit.

The spectrum of activity is the same as that of ACE inhibitors, but the main advantage is that these drugs do not prevent the breakdown of bradykinin, so cough does not occur as a side effect.

Diuretics

Loop diuretics, such as furosemide and thiazide diuretics such as bendrofluazide or metolazone (Fig. 15.6) have an important role in salt and water excretion. They provide symptomatic relief, but have no effect on mortality in heart failure.

Aldosterone antagonists

Spironolactone is a weak diuretic that acts by blocking aldosterone receptors in the distal convoluted tubule. Aldosterone promotes sodium retention and potassium excretion; it also has a number of unfavourable extrarenal effects, including sympathetic

Fig. 15.6 Site of action and side-effects of different diuretics

Examples	Site of action	Side-effects
Loop diuretics: furosemide (frusemide), bumetanide, ethacrynic acid	Thick ascending loop of Henle	Ototoxicity with ethacrynic acid; hypokalaemia; exacerbation of gout
Thiazide diuretics: bendroflumethiazide (bendrofluazide), hydrochlorthiazide, metolazone	Distal convoluted tubule	Hyperglycaemia, gout, elevated triglycerides/LDL, hypokalaemia, hyponatraemia
Potassium-sparing diuretics: amiloride, spironolactone	Collecting duct and distal convoluted tubule	Hyperkalaemia – use with caution with ACE inhibitors

ACE, angiotensin-converting enzyme; LDL, low-density lipoprotein.

stimulation, parasympathetic inhibition, vascular damage and impairment of arterial compliance, all of which adversely affect cardiac function. It is thought that spironolactone potentiates the action of ACE inhibitors by suppressing aldosterone activity and its adverse effects. Patients with severe heart failure receiving both drugs have a 30% lower mortality rate than patients receiving placebo. Caution is needed, however, as both medications cause potassium retention, which can reach dangerous levels. It is, therefore, crucial to measure serum electrolytes regularly. Other side effects of spironolactone include gynaecomastia and breast pain in men.

Eplerenone is licensed in patients post myocardial infarction who have clinical signs of heart failure and LV systolic impairment, and has been shown to confer a mortality benefit in this group.

Patients with heart failure should be advised to monitor their weight at home, in conjunction with their degree of breathlessness on exertion. If these parameters increase, the dose of diuretic can be adjusted by the patient. If the opposite occurs and the patient is more dehydrated than usual (weight loss) then diuretic dose can be reduced as necessary. This is especially important if the patient has diarrhoea, as renal failure can ensue, if combined treatment with several drugs (for example, furosemide, spironolactone and ACE inhibitor) is continued in this setting.

β-Blockers

The negative inotropic effect of β-blockers has made their use in cardiac failure extremely rare until recently. Indeed, medical students have always been reminded that cardiac failure is a contraindication to the use of β-blockers.

As always in medicine one can never say never, and it seems that β-blockers are in fact an effective treatment option in cardiac failure. As mentioned on pp. 121–3, there is a high circulating rate of catecholamines in cardiac failure. There is also a downregulation of β-receptors in response to this (perhaps the heart's way of protecting itself from the tachycardia and increased metabolic rate that result from sympathetic stimulation). Recent trials of metoprolol, bisoprolol and carvedilol have shown benefit in their use in cardiac failure. This could be for a number of reasons:

- Reduction in myocardial oxygen demand and ischaemia
- Decreased incidence of arrhythmias
- Peripheral vasodilatation with non-selective β-blockers that have some α-blockade as well
- Antioxidant effects (carvedilol).

Carvedilol, a non-selective β-blocker with α-blocking activity, has been shown to reduce mortality rates in chronic heart failure by over 30%.

β-Blockers must be introduced with care to patients who have heart failure because they may cause the patient's symptoms to deteriorate. There is still no evidence to suggest that they have efficacy in patients who have severe heart failure (i.e. dyspnoea at rest) or acute heart failure.

Patients who have heart failure should be stabilized with other drugs before being prescribed β-blockers.

Nitrates

The nitrates (e.g. isosorbide mononitrate and isosorbide dinitrate) are veno- and arteriolar dilators and, therefore, act by reducing load. Intravenous nitrates are useful in the treatment of the acutely sick patient with cardiac failure. Oral nitrates may provide some symptomatic relief in chronic cardiac failure. The combination of nitrates and hydralazine has been shown to reduce the mortality rate of cardiac failure.

Digoxin

Digoxin is a cardiac glycoside. It inhibits the sodium/potassium pump on the sarcolemmal and cell membranes. This adenosine triphosphate (ATP)-dependent pump plays a role in transporting calcium out of the cell. Its inhibition, therefore, prevents this, resulting in increased intracellular calcium concentration, which in cardiac muscle results in a positive inotropic effect.

In AV node tissue the effect of an increased calcium concentration is to prolong the refractory period and decrease AV node conduction velocity, so slowing AV node conduction of the cardiac impulse – a negative chronotropic effect.

It is generally accepted that digoxin is an extremely useful drug in patients with atrial fibrillation and cardiac failure, but that there is no evidence to suggest that its use as an antifailure agent alone is effective in reducing mortality rates.

Pharmacokinetics

Digoxin has a half-life of 24–36 h and it takes 3–4 weeks to reach a steady plasma level after oral loading. Intravenous loading speeds this up slightly because the time taken for absorption in the gut is bypassed; 40% of digoxin in the blood is protein bound.

Excretion is predominantly renal (10% excreted in the stools) and digoxin should not be used in renal failure. In mild renal impairment the dose is reduced.

Side effects

Plasma levels of digoxin should be monitored and maintained at between 1 and 2 ng/mL. Blood is taken 6 h after an oral dose. Digoxin toxicity is more likely in patients who:

- have renal failure
- are hypokalaemic – digoxin competes with potassium for binding to the sodium/potassium ATPase
- are taking amiodarone or verapamil (which displace digoxin from protein binding sites), erythromycin (which prevents inactivation of digoxin by gut bacteria) or captopril (which reduces renal clearance of digoxin).

Signs of digoxin toxicity are:

- bradycardia, AV block and sinus arrest
- nausea and vomiting
- xanthopsia (yellow discoloration of visualized objects).

Hydralazine

Hydralazine is a potent vasodilator, predominantly of arterioles; therefore, it reduces load, which acts to improve cardiac function. Side effects include flushing and a lupus-like syndrome.

Cardiac resynchronization treatment

Approximately one-third of patients with heart failure have an abnormality in the conduction pathway. This manifests as prolongation of the QRS duration (>120 ms) and results in parts of the ventricle being activated in an asynchronous manner. Consequently, relaxation in diastole is also asynchronous with parts of the ventricle relaxing while other parts are still contracting. In normal hearts, the effects of this are probably unnoticeable. However, in dilated, poorly functioning hearts it has a significant effect in reducing stroke volume and cardiac output and can lead to mitral regurgitation. Resynchronization treatment involves implanting a pacemaker to activate the ventricles in a synchronous manner to improve relaxation and ventricular filling, and subsequently stroke volume and cardiac output. New pacemakers are biventricular devices in which three pacing leads are used in the right atrium, right ventricle and left ventricle (via the coronary sinus). This is thought to simulate normal physiological activation of the ventricles. Clinical trials have shown that the use of such devices significantly improves patients' quality of life, the amount of exercise they are able to perform and, more recently, a mortality benefit has been demonstrated.

Further reading

ACC/AHA Committee and task force members 2005 Guidelines for the evaluation and management of chronic heart failure in the adult: executive summary. *Circulation* **112**: e154–e235

Cleland J, Daubert J-C, Erdmann E et al 2005 The effect of Cardiac Resynchronization on Morbidity and Mortality in Heart Failure (CARE-HF). *N Engl J Med* **352**: 1539–49

Foody J M, Farrell M H, Krumholz H M 2002 Beta-blocker therapy in heart failure: scientific review. *JAMA* **287**: 883–9

Gibbs C R, Jackson G, Lip G Y H 2000 ABC of heart failure. Non-drug management. *BMJ* **320**: 366–9

Heart Outcomes Prevention Evaluation Study Investigators (HOPE) 2000 Effects of ramipril on cardiovascular and microvascular outcomes in people with diabetes mellitus. *Lancet* **355**: 253–9

Jackson G, Gibbs C R, Davies M K, Lip G Y H 2000 ABC of heart failure. Pathophysiology. *BMJ* **320**: 167–70

Millane T, Jackson G, Gibbs C R, Lip G Y H 2000 ABC of heart failure. Acute and chronic management strategies. *BMJ* **320**: 559–62

Pitt B, Zannad F, Remme W J et al 1999 The effect of spironolactone on morbidity and mortality in patients with severe heart failure. *N Engl J Med* **341**: 709–17

The cardiomyopathies

Objectives

By the end of this chapter you should:

- be able to list the causes of dilated cardiomyopathy
- know the different types of cardiomyopathy
- understand the principles of investigation of patients with cardiomyopathy
- be able to carry out a risk stratification of patients with hypertrophic cardiomyopathy.

DEFINITION OF CARDIOMYOPATHY

Cardiomyopathy is heart muscle disease, often of unknown cause. Ischaemic cardiomyopathy is heart failure due to underlying coronary artery disease and is discussed elsewhere. There are four types (Fig. 16.1):

1. Dilated cardiomyopathy
2. Hypertrophic cardiomyopathy
3. Restrictive cardiomyopathy
4. Arrhythmogenic right-ventricular cardiomyopathy.

DILATED CARDIOMYOPATHY

The heart is dilated and has impaired function. The coronary arteries are normal. Probable causes of dilated cardiomyopathy include:

- alcohol
- viral infection (echovirus, coxsackievirus, and enteroviruses most likely)
- untreated hypertension
- autoimmune disease
- thyrotoxicosis
- drugs (cocaine, doxorubicin, cyclophosphamide or lead)
- haemochromatosis
- acquired immune deficiency syndrome (AIDS).

Clinical features

Progressive biventricular cardiac failure leads to:

- fatigue
- dyspnoea
- peripheral oedema
- ascites.

Other complications secondary to the progressive dilatation of the ventricles include:

- mural thrombi with systemic or pulmonary embolization
- dilatation of the tricuspid and mitral valve rings leading to functional valve regurgitation
- atrial fibrillation
- ventricular tachyarrhythmias and sudden death.

Investigation

Investigations to aid diagnosis are listed below.

Chest radiography

This may show:

- enlarged cardiac shadow
- signs of pulmonary oedema (upper lobe blood diversion or interstitial shadowing at the bases)
- pleural effusions.

Electrocardiography

Electrocardiography may highlight:

- tachycardia
- poor R wave progression across the chest leads
- conduction delay such as left bundle branch block.

Fig. 16.1 Different types of cardiomyopathy. AV, aortic valve; HCM, hypertrophic cardiomyopathy; LA, left atrium; LV, left ventricle; MR, mitral regurgitation; MV, mitral valve.

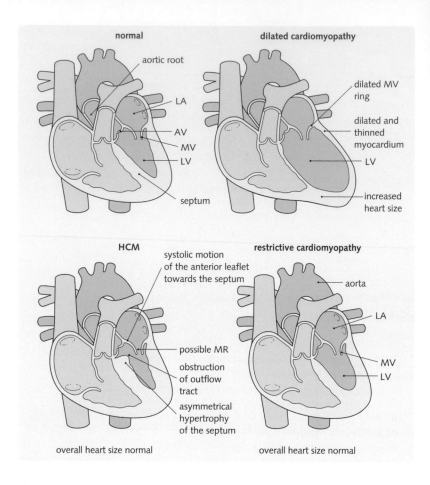

Echocardiography

Points to consider with echocardiography include:

- can the dilated ventricles be easily visualized?
- can the regurgitant valves be seen?

Occasionally, intracardiac thrombus may be seen. Transthoracic echocardiography is not a reliable method for diagnosing this, but it can be accurately diagnosed by transoesophageal echocardiography.

Cardiac catheterization

This is important to exclude coronary artery disease (the most common cause of ventricular dysfunction).

Magnetic resonance imaging

This is an excellent non-invasive tool for assessment of patients with cardiomyopathy, and late enhancement with gadolinium can provide useful information about the aetiology and prognosis.

Blood tests

Viral titres may be useful and also thyroid function tests.

Management

The management plan follows four basic steps (the same applies for any other case of cardiac failure):

1. Search for and treat any underlying cause (e.g. stop alcohol)
2. Treat cardiac failure (diuretics, ACE inhibitors or β-blockers)
3. Treat any arrhythmias (β-blockers, digoxin or amiodarone for atrial fibrillation, or amiodarone for ventricular arrhythmias)
4. Consider anticoagulation with warfarin to prevent mural thrombi.

After optimization of medical therapy, devicetherapy should be considered (see pp. 105, 132). Cardiac transplantation may also be a treatment option.

HYPERTROPHIC CARDIOMYOPATHY

This disorder is characterized by asymmetrical hypertrophy of the cardiac septum – the interventricular septum is hypertrophied compared to the free wall of the left ventricle.

The inheritance in most cases is autosomal dominant with equal sex distribution. The genetic abnormality is the subject of much current research and different genes may be involved in different families.

The myocytes of the left ventricle are abnormally thick when examined microscopically and their layout is disorganized (myocardial disarray). This makes left-ventricular filling more difficult than normal and grossly disordered. There is left-ventricular outflow tract obstruction in many cases, and this condition is often called hypertrophic obstructive cardiomyopathy (HOCM).

Clinical features

There are four main symptoms:

1. Angina (even in the absence of coronary artery disease) – due to the increased oxygen demands of the hypertrophied muscle
2. Palpitations – there is an increased incidence of atrial fibrillation and ventricular arrhythmias in this condition
3. Syncope and sudden death – which may be due to left-ventricular outflow tract obstruction by the hypertrophied septum or to a ventricular arrhythmia
4. Dyspnoea – due to the stiff left ventricle, which leads to a high end-diastolic pressure and can, therefore, lead to pulmonary oedema.

It is highly unlikely that you will be presented with a patient who has HCM to diagnose as a short case in finals, but you may be presented with such a patient as a long case. The signs (Fig. 16.2) to watch for are:

- Jerky peripheral pulse – the second rise palpable in the pulse is due to the rise in left-ventricular pressure as the left ventricle attempts to overcome the outflow tract obstruction.
- Double apical beat – the stiff left ventricle causes raised left ventricular end-diastolic pressure. The atrial contraction is, therefore, very forceful to fill the left ventricle. It is this atrial impulse that can be felt in addition to the left-ventricular contraction that gives this classical sign.

- Systolic thrill – felt at the left lower sternal edge.
- Systolic murmur – crescendo and decrescendo in nature, and best heard between the apex and the left lower sternal edge.

It can be difficult to differentiate between HCM and aortic stenosis on examination. Use the following features to help:

- Pulse – slow rising in aortic stenosis, jerky or with a normal upstroke in HCM.
- Second heart sound – reduced in intensity in significant aortic stenosis
- Thrill and murmur – both found in the second right intercostal space in aortic stenosis and at the left lower sternal edge in HCM
- Variation of the murmur with Valsalva manoeuvre – this does not occur in aortic stenosis, but the murmur of HCM is increased because the volume of the left ventricle is reduced by the manoeuvre and, therefore, the outflow obstruction worsens.

Remember that the outflow obstruction of aortic stenosis is fixed and is present throughout systole, whereas the obstruction of HCM is often absent at the start of systole and worsens as the ventricle empties.

Diagnosis and investigations

Electrocardiography

This is usually abnormal in HCM. The most common abnormalities are T wave and ST segment abnormalities; the signs of left-ventricular hypertrophy may also be present.

Continuous ambulatory electrocardiography

The presence of ventricular arrhythmias is common in patients who have HCM and is a cause of sudden death. It is thought that the presence of ventricular arrhythmias on an ambulatory ECG monitor is a risk factor for sudden death and that an antiarrhythmic agent should be commenced. These tests are usually performed as part of a yearly screening programme for these patients.

Fig. 16.2 Important clinical signs in hypertrophic obstructive cardiomyopathy. AV, aortic valve; JVP, jugular venous pressure; LV, left ventricle.

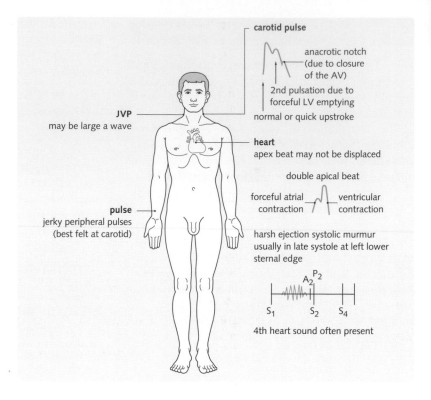

Echocardiography

This is the most useful investigation because it confirms the diagnosis and can be used to assess the degree of outflow tract obstruction.

Characteristic echocardiography findings include:

- asymmetrical hypertrophy of the septum
- abnormal systolic anterior motion of the anterior leaflet of the mitral valve
- left-ventricular outflow tract obstruction.

Prognosis

Children who are diagnosed when they are under 14 years of age have a poor prognosis and a high incidence of sudden death. Adults have a better prognosis, but they also have a higher mortality rate than the general population. Another outcome is progressive cardiac failure with cardiac dilatation.

Management

Drug management

As with aortic stenosis, vasodilators should be avoided because they worsen the gradient across the obstruction. Therefore, patients who have HCM should not receive nitrates.

β-Blockers (β-adrenoceptor antagonists) are used because their negative inotropic effect acts to decrease the contractility of the hypertrophied septum and reduce the outflow tract obstruction. They also increase ventricular filling time and reduce incidence of arrhymias.

Antiarrhythmic agents are important in patients who have ventricular and atrial arrhythmias. Patients who have atrial fibrillation should be cardioverted as soon as possible (patients who have a high left ventricular end-diastolic pressure rely on the atrial impulse to fill the left ventricle effectively).

Patients should be advised that first-degree relatives should be screened with a transthoracic echocardiogram in cases of dilated or hypertrophic cardiomyopathy as these are often hereditary.

Device therapy

Dual chamber pacing may reduce the outflow tract gradient, but objective evidence of benefit is poor.

An implantable cardioverter defibrillator (ICD) should be considered in patients at high risk of sudden cardiac death (see box below).

Percutaneous treatment (alcohol septal ablation)

In suitable cases, alcohol can be injected down the septal branch of the left anterior descending coronary artery, causing necrosis of the myocardial tissue that gives rise to the obstruction.

Surgery

Surgery is used only when all other treatments have failed. A myomectomy is performed on the abnormal septum. This is the treatment of choice if other cardiac structural abnormalities need surgical correction.

Features that increase the risk of sudden cardiac death are:

- Genetic: family history of sudden cardiac death or genetic mutation associated with high risk
- Clinical: documented ventricular arrhythmia or history of syncope
- Haemodynamic: exercise-related fall in blood pressure or high pressure gradient across LV outflow tract
- Structural: extreme LV hypertrophy (>3 mm).

RESTRICTIVE CARDIOMYOPATHY

This is an uncommon cause of cardiomyopathy in developed countries. The ventricular walls are excessively stiff and impede ventricular filling; therefore, end-diastolic pressure is increased. The systolic function of the ventricle is often normal.

Presentation is identical to that of constrictive pericarditis, but the two must be differentiated because pericardial constriction can be treated with surgery.

Possible causes of restrictive cardiomyopathy include:

- storage diseases (e.g. glycogen storage diseases)
- infiltrative diseases (e.g. amyloidosis, sarcoidosis)
- scleroderma
- endomyocardial diseases (e.g. endomyocardial fibrosis, hypereosinophilic syndrome or carcinoid)

Clinical features

The main features are:

- dyspnoea and fatigue due to poor cardiac output
- peripheral oedema and ascites
- elevated jugular venous pressure with a positive Kussmaul's sign (increase in jugular venous pressure during inspiration).

Management

There is no specific treatment and the condition usually progresses towards death relatively quickly; most patients do not survive beyond 10 years after diagnosis.

ARRHYTHMOGENIC RIGHT-VENTRICULAR CARDIOMYOPATHY

This is a relatively rare condition that is thought to arise from fibrofatty replacement of the right ventricular wall. The main problem that this causes is heart rhythm disturbance ranging from ectopic beats to sustained ventricular arrhythmias and even sudden cardiac death. There may also be impairment of right-ventricular function.

Patients present with palpitations, syncope, heart failure or sudden death.

Diagnosis is best made with cardiac MRI if clinical suspicion arises.

There is no curative treatment, so management is aimed at preventing complications. This includes the use of ACE inhibitors and diuretics for the treatment of heart failure, antiarrhythmic agents and consideration of ICD implantation in patients at high risk of sudden cardiac death.

Further reading

Kushwaha S S, Fallon J T, Fuster V 1997 Restrictive cardiomyopathy. *N Engl J Med* **336**: 267–76

Oakley C Dec 1997 Aetiology, diagnosis, investigation, and management of the cardiomyopathies. *BMJ* **315**: 1520–4

Pennell D J 2002 Arrhythmogenic right ventricular cardiomyopathy; www.escardio.org/knowledge/cardiology_practice/ejournal_vol1/Vol1_no7.htm

Spirito P, Seidman C E, McKenna W J, Maron B J 1997 The management of hypertrophic cardiomyopathy. *N Engl J Med* **336**: 775–85

Wynne S, Braunwald E 2001 The cardiomyopathies and myocarditides. In: Braunwald E, Zipes D P (eds) Heart disease: a textbook of cardiovascular medicine, 6th edn. W B Saunders & Co, Elsevier

The pericardium forms a strong protective sac around the heart. It is composed of an outer fibrous and an inner serosal layer with approximately 50 mL of pericardial fluid between these in the healthy state.

ACUTE PERICARDITIS

Acute pericarditis is caused by inflammation of the pericardium (Fig. 17.1).

Clinical features

History

The chest pain of acute pericarditis is usually central or left-sided pain that is sharp in nature and relieved by sitting forwards. Aggravating factors include lying supine and coughing.

Dyspnoea may be caused by the pain of deep inspiration or the haemodynamic effects of an associated pericardial effusion.

Examination

The patient may have a fever and tachycardia.

A pericardial friction rub may be heard on auscultation of the heart. This is a high-pitched scratching sound (therefore, heard best with the diaphragm). It characteristically varies with time and may appear and disappear from one examination to the next. It sounds closer to the ears than a murmur.

Investigation

Blood tests

These will provide evidence of active inflammation – raised white cell count, erythrocyte sedimentation rate (ESR) and C-reactive protein (CRP), and also clues about the underlying cause. The following blood tests are appropriate:

- Full blood count
- ESR and CRP
- Urea, creatinine and electrolytes
- Viral titres in the acute and convalescent phase (3 weeks later); also urine and faecal samples for viral studies and a Paul-Bunnell test
- Blood cultures (at least three)
- Autoantibody titres (e.g. antinuclear antibodies and rheumatoid factor)
- Cardiac enzymes and cardiac troponin T/troponin I – these may be elevated, suggesting that the inflammatory process involves the myocardium (myopericarditis).

Electrocardiography

Superficial myocardial injury caused by pericarditis results in characteristic ECG changes (Fig. 17.2):

- Concave ST segment elevation is usually present in all leads, except AVR and V1.
- Subsequently, a few days later, the ST segments return to normal and T wave flattening occurs and may even become inverted.
- Finally, all of the changes resolve and the ECG trace returns to normal (this may take several weeks or, if the inflammation persists, may remain for many months).

Chest radiography

This is normal in most cases of uncomplicated acute pericarditis; however, a number of changes are possible:

Fig. 17.1 Causes of acute pericarditis

Cause	Examples/comment
Viral infection	Coxsackie virus A and B, echovirus, Epstein–Barr virus, HIV
Bacterial infection	Pneumococci, staphylococci, Gram-negative organisms, *Neisseria meningitidis*, *N. gonorrhoeae*
Fungal infection	Histoplasmosis, candidal infection
Other infections	Tuberculosis
Acute MI	Occurs in up to 25% of patients between 12 h and 6 days after infarction
Uraemia	Usually a haemorrhagic pericarditis, which can rapidly lead to cardiac tamponade; uraemic pericarditis is an indication for haemodialysis
Autoimmune disease	Acute rheumatic fever, SLE, rheumatoid arthritis, scleroderma
Other causes	Neoplastic disease, other inflammatory diseases, e.g. sarcoidosis, Whipple's disease, Behçet's syndrome, Dressler's syndrome

Fig. 17.2 ECG changes of pericarditis. Note the concave or saddle-shaped ST elevation seen in all leads except AVR.

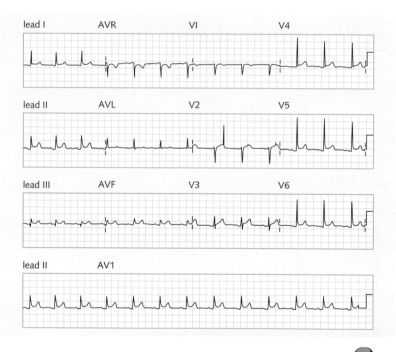

- A pericardial effusion may develop and if large will result in enlargement of the cardiac shadow, which assumes a globular shape.
- Pleural effusions may also be seen.

A dissecting thoracic aortic aneurysm may occasionally present as acute pericarditis or a pericardial effusion. Therefore, be careful to look for a widened mediastinum on the chest radiograph and if this is suspicious a computed tomography scan of the chest or trans-oesophageal echo (TOE) should be performed to avoid missing this diagnosis.

Echocardiography

This is the best investigation for confirming the presence of a pericardial effusion. In uncomplicated acute pericarditis, however, the echocardiogram may be normal.

Management

Any treatable underlying cause should of course be sought and treated appropriately. Most cases of pericarditis are viral or idiopathic. The main aims of management are, therefore, analgesia and bed rest. Non-steroidal anti-inflammatory agents are the most effective for this condition. Occasionally a short course of oral corticosteroids is required.

A pericardial effusion may be present. If large or causing tamponade this can be drained. Analysis of the effusion may provide clues about the underlying cause of the pericarditis.

DRESSLER'S SYNDROME

Dressler's syndrome is a syndrome of fever, pericarditis and pleurisy occurring more than 1 week after a cardiac operation or myocardial infarction (MI). It can occur only if the pericardium has been exposed to the blood. Antibodies form against the pericardial antigens and then attack the pericardium in a type III autoimmune reaction.

Patients present with fever, malaise and chest pain. They exhibit the classic signs of acute pericarditis; they may also have arthritis. Cardiac tamponade is not uncommon.

Chest radiography shows pleural effusions. Echocardiography may reveal a pericardial effusion.

Initial management consists of non-steroidal anti-inflammatory agents and aspirin; corticosteroids may be added if the symptoms persist.

CHRONIC CONSTRICTIVE PERICARDITIS

Chronic constrictive pericarditis occurs when the pericardium becomes fibrosed and thickened and eventually restricts the filling of the heart during diastole. Causes are listed in Fig. 17.3.

Fig. 17.3 Causes of chronic constrictive pericarditis

- Viral infection
- Tuberculosis
- Mediastinal radiotherapy
- Mediastinal malignancy
- Autoimmune disease

Note that any cause of acute pericarditis can persist and lead to chronic constrictive pericarditis. The diseases listed here, however, seem to be the most common causes.

Clinical features

The restricted filling of all four chambers of the heart results in low-output failure.

Initially, the right-sided component is more marked, resulting in a high venous pressure and hepatic congestion.

Later, left-ventricular failure (LVF) becomes apparent with dyspnoea and orthopnoea.

Examination

On examination, the signs of RVF and LVF are evident, but the ventricles are not enlarged.

The single most important feature in the examination of such a patient is the jugular venous pressure (JVP), which is elevated. Kussmaul's sign – an increase in the JVP during inspiration – may be evident.

Another important feature of the JVP is a rapid x and y descent. This is an important differential diagnostic point when trying to exclude tamponade. There is no such feature in tamponade.

The heart sounds are often soft. Atrial fibrillation is common.

Investigation

Blood tests are carried out to exclude a possible underlying cause (e.g. leucocytosis in infection, viral titres).

On chest radiography the heart size is normal. There may be signs of a neoplasm or tuberculosis. Pleural effusions are not uncommon. Tuberculous pericarditis may be associated with radiographically visible calcification.

Echocardiography shows good left-ventricular function.

Cardiac catheterization is diagnostic because it shows the classical pattern of raised left and right end-diastolic pressures with normal left-ventricular function on the ventriculogram.

Management

The only definitive treatment is pericardectomy.

Antituberculous therapy may be required if the underlying cause is tuberculosis and should be continued for 1 year.

PERICARDIAL EFFUSION

A pericardial effusion is an accumulation of fluid in the pericardial space.

Cardiac tamponade describes the condition where a pericardial effusion increases the intrapericardial pressure such that it leads to haemodynamic compromise.

Causes

Causes of pericardial effusion (Fig. 17.4) include:

- acute pericarditis (see Fig. 17.1)
- MI with ventricular wall rupture
- chest trauma
- cardiac surgery
- aortic dissection
- neoplasia.

Clinical features

A pericardial effusion may remain asymptomatic, even if very large, if it accumulates gradually. As much as 2 L of fluid can be accommodated without an increase in intrapericardial pressure if it accumulates slowly, but as little as 100 mL can cause tamponade if it appears suddenly.

Fig. 17.4 Causes of a pericardial effusion

Type of effusion	Examples
Transudate (<30 g/L protein)	Congestive cardiac failure, hypoalbuminaemia
Exudate (>30 g/L protein)	Infection (viral, bacterial or fungal), postmyocardial infarction, malignancy (e.g. local invasion of lung tumour), systemic lupus erythematosus, Dressler's syndrome
Haemorrhagic	Uraemia, aortic dissection, trauma and postcardiac surgery

History

The only symptoms produced by a large chronic effusion may be a dull ache in the chest or dysphagia from compression of the oesophagus.

If cardiac tamponade is present, however, the patient may complain of dyspnoea, abdominal swelling (due to ascites) and peripheral oedema.

Examination

The important examination findings in a patient who has tamponade are:

- low blood pressure
- pulse – tachycardia with low volume pulse, and may be pulsus paradoxus (where there is an exaggerated reduction of the pulse >10 mmHg during inspiration)
- soft heart sounds
- low urine output.
- raised jugular venous pressure.

Possible mechanisms for pulsus paradoxus

These are:

- increased venous return during inspiration filling the right heart and restricting left-ventricular filling, because the pericardium forms a rigid sac with only limited space within it
- downward movement of the diaphragm causing traction on the pericardium and tightening it further (this theory is not widely supported).

Investigation

Electrocardiography

A pericardial effusion results in the production of small voltage complexes with variable axis (electrical alternans is caused by the movement of the heart within the fluid).

On chest radiography the heart may appear large and globular.

Echocardiography reveals the pericardial effusion. Right-ventricular diastolic collapse is a classical echocardiographic sign of tamponade.

Management

The pericardial effusion should be drained if causing haemodynamic compromise or if there is doubt about the underlying cause. If the patient is in cardiogenic shock due to tamponade an emergency pericardial needle aspiration may be performed followed by formal drainage once the patient has been resuscitated.

Both techniques involve insertion of the drain or needle just below the xiphisternum and advancing it at 45° to the skin in the direction of the patient's left shoulder. The fluid should be sent for cytology, microscopy, culture and biochemical analysis of protein content.

Long-term treatment depends on the underlying cause.

Following drainage of pericardial effusion and discharge from hospital, patients should be made aware of the symptoms they will experience should the effusion reaccumulate, in order that they should seek medical help. These symptoms include lethargy, shortness of breath, abdominal swelling and peripheral oedema.

Further reading

Spodick D H 2003 Acute cardiac tamponade. *N Engl J Med* **349**: 684–90

Sagristà-Sauleda J, Angel J, Permanyer-Miralda G, Soler-Soler J 1999 Long-term follow-up of idiopathic chronic pericardial effusion. *N Engl J Med* **341**: 2054–9

Sagristà-Sauleda J, Angel J, Sánchez A, Permanyer-Miralda G, Soler-Soler J 2004 Effusive-constrictive pericarditis. *N Engl J Med* **350**: 469–75

Objectives

By the end of this chapter you should:

- understand the natural history, diagnosis and consequences of rheumatic fever
- be able to list the causes of mitral and aortic valve disease
- be able to recognize the clinical signs and evaluate the severity of heart valve disease
- appreciate the effects on normal physiology of mitral and aortic valve stenosis and regurgitation
- be able to remember the treatment modalities for different valve lesions
- be aware of different types of heart valve prosthesis.

This topic is touched on in Chapters 6 and 23, but it is covered here in more detail.

Valve lesions are a common short-case question both in finals and in the membership examination. It is possible to learn valve disease parrot fashion – once you know it you will not forget it again so it will be time well spent (Fig. 18.1). Alternatively, familiarity with the physiology (see *Crash course: cardiovascular system*) will enable you to understand the features of valve disease from first principles.

RHEUMATIC FEVER

As mentioned in Chapters 8 and 19, rheumatic fever is much less common in the developed world than in developing countries due to better social conditions and antibiotic therapy, and also because of a reduction in the virulence of β-haemolytic streptococcus. It is still a major problem in the developing world, where it is responsible for more heart disease than any other single disease.

Causes

Rheumatic fever is caused by a group A streptococcal pharyngeal infection. It occurs 2–3 weeks later in a small percentage of children aged 5–15 years. It is an antibody-mediated autoimmune response (type II hypersensitivity) and occurs where antibodies directed against bacterial cell membrane antigens cross-react and cause multiorgan disease.

Clinical features

Diagnosis is entirely clinical. Diagnosis based on the Duckett-Jones criteria requires evidence of preceding β-haemolytic streptococcal infection (e.g. increased antistreptolysin O titres) plus one major criterion or two minor criteria. Major criteria are:

- carditis – involves all layers (pancarditis) and is usually asymptomatic
- arthritis – a migrating polyarthritis affecting the larger joints
- Sydenham's chorea – usually occurs months after the initial disease and characterized by involuntary movements of the face and mouth due to inflammation of the caudate nucleus
- erythema marginatum – seen mainly on the trunk; the rash has raised red edges and a clear centre and the shape of the lesions changes with time
- nodules – pea-sized subcutaneous nodules on the extensor surfaces (painless).

Minor criteria are:

- fever
- previous rheumatic fever
- raised erythrocyte sedimentation rate (ESR) or C-reactive protein (CRP)
- long PR interval
- arthralgia.

Fig. 18.1 Valve lesions and their abbreviations

Valve involved	Lesion	Abbreviation
Mitral valve	Mitral stenosis	MS
	Mitral regurgitation	MR
	Floppy (prolapsing) mitral valve	MVP
Aortic valve	Aortic stenosis	AS
	Aortic regurgitation	AR
Tricuspid valve	Tricuspid regurgitation	TR
	Tricuspid stenosis	TS
Pulmonary valve	Pulmonary stenosis	PS
	Pulmonary regurgitation	PR

Investigations

Blood tests reveal raised inflammatory markers (ESR and CRP) and rising antistreptolysin O (ASO) titres when taken 2 weeks apart. The throat swab may be positive.

Management

Treatment with high-dose benzylpenicillin is started immediately to eradicate the causative organism. Anti-inflammatory agents are given to suppress the autoimmune response. Salicylates are effective. Corticosteroids are used if there is any carditis. Long-term follow-up is required and any patients who have resulting valve damage need prophylactic antibiotics to prevent infective endocarditis.

> Acute rheumatic fever is not common in the developed world, but it is a good idea to have knowledge of this disease because there are still many elderly people suffering the after-effects of a childhood infection. It is also important to recognize and treat acute rheumatic fever promptly.

MITRAL STENOSIS

Causes

The most common cause of mitral stenosis (MS) is rheumatic fever (Fig. 18.2). Other causes are rare:

- Congenital: isolated lesion or associated with an atrial septal defect (Lutembacher's syndrome)
- Malignant – carcinoid
- Systemic lupus erythematosus
- Mucopolysaccharidoses, e.g. Hurler's syndrome (causing glycoprotein deposition on the mitral leaflets)
- Endocardial fibroelastosis spreading onto the valve.

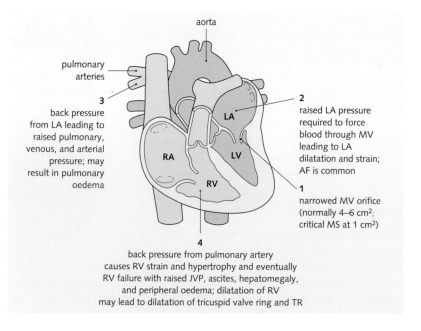

Fig. 18.2 Pathophysiology of mitral stenosis. AF, atrial fibrillation; LA, left atrium; LV, left ventricle; JVP, jugular venous pressure; MV, mitral valve; RA, right atrium; RV, right ventricle; TR, tricuspid regurgitation.

aorta

pulmonary arteries

3 back pressure from LA leading to raised pulmonary, venous, and arterial pressure; may result in pulmonary oedema

2 raised LA pressure required to force blood through MV leading to LA dilatation and strain; AF is common

1 narrowed MV orifice (normally 4–6 cm²; critical MS at 1 cm²)

4 back pressure from pulmonary artery causes RV strain and hypertrophy and eventually RV failure with raised JVP, ascites, hepatomegaly, and peripheral oedema; dilatation of RV may lead to dilatation of tricuspid valve ring and TR

Other conditions may mimic mitral stenosis by causing obstruction of inflow to the left ventricle. These include left atrial myxoma, left atrial thrombus and hypertrophic cardiomyopathy.

Rheumatic fever causes fusion of the cusps and commissures, and thickening of the cusps, which then become immobile and stenosed in a fish-mouth configuration. An immobile valve cannot close properly and is, therefore, often regurgitant as well.

Clinical features

The main presenting features of mitral stenosis are:

- dyspnoea – this may be due to pulmonary hypertension or pulmonary oedema. Patients who have mitral stenosis have an increased incidence of chest infections, which may cause dyspnoea.
- haemoptysis – there is an increased incidence of pulmonary vein and alveolar capillary rupture
- palpitations – atrial fibrillation is common in this condition (due to enlargement of the left atrium) and may cause palpitations, which are often accompanied by a sudden worsening in the dyspnoea because the loss of the atrial contraction (upon which the heart has become dependent) causes a considerable reduction in cardiac output
- systemic emboli – a recognized complication of atrial fibrillation.

Symptoms that are secondary to effects of left atrial enlargement include:

- hoarseness due to stretching of the recurrent laryngeal nerve
- dysphagia due to oesophageal compression
- left lung collapse due to compression of the left main bronchus.

Examination

The principal clinical findings (Fig. 18.3) are:

- loud first heart sound (S_1), due to the mitral valve slamming shut at the beginning of ventricular systole
- a tapping apex beat that is not displaced
- an opening snap after the second heart sound (S_2) followed by a low rumbling mid-diastolic murmur, heard best at the apex with the patient on his or her left side and in expiration. If you have not listened in exactly this way you cannot exclude MS.
- a presystolic accentuation of the mid-diastolic murmur, if the patient is in sinus rhythm; this is absent if the patient has atrial fibrillation. Severity is related to the duration, not the intensity, of the mid-diastolic murmur
- loud and palpable pulmonary component of the second heart sound (P_2), if pulmonary

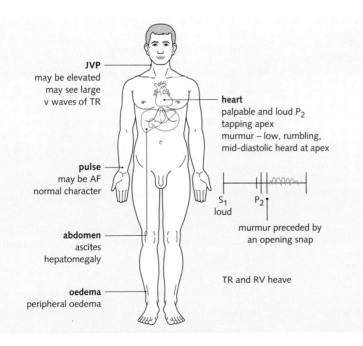

Fig. 18.3 Clinical findings in patients who have mitral stenosis. AF, atrial fibrillation; S_1, first heart sound; P_2, pulmonary component of second heart sound; RV, right ventricle; TR, tricuspid regurgitation.

JVP
may be elevated
may see large
v waves of TR

heart
palpable and loud P_2
tapping apex
murmur – low, rumbling,
mid-diastolic heard at apex

pulse
may be AF
normal character

S_1
loud

P_2

murmur preceded by
an opening snap

abdomen
ascites
hepatomegaly

TR and RV heave

oedema
peripheral oedema

hypertension has developed, and there may be a right ventricular heave. Tricuspid regurgitation may be present.

> Mitral stenosis is a difficult murmur to hear. It is, therefore, vital to listen for the murmur correctly (i.e. with the patient on his or her left side in full expiration).

Investigations

Investigations that may aid diagnosis include the following:

Electrocardiography

Atrial fibrillation may be seen. P mitrale is another feature and is only seen in sinus rhythm. The P wave in lead II is abnormally long (0.12 s) and may have an 'M' shape.

Chest radiography

This shows the enlarged left atrium. The carina may be widely split. The mitral valve itself may be calcified and, therefore, visible. There may be prominent pulmonary vessels.

Echocardiography

The mitral valve can be visualized and the cross-sectional area measured. This can also be estimated using Doppler measurements. Pulmonary hypertension can also be evaluated.

Cardiac catheterization

This is performed on most patients before valve replacement to exclude any coexistent coronary artery disease and evaluate any mitral regurgitation that may be present.

Management

Medical management

Medical treatment of MS may consist of:

- digoxin or a small dose of a β-blocker (β-adrenoceptor antagonist) – may be used to treat atrial fibrillation, and by prolonging diastole allow the left ventricle more time to fill
- direct current (DC) cardioversion – may be successful in patients who have atrial fibrillation of recent onset, but only if they have been fully anticoagulated for at least 4 weeks
- anticoagulation with warfarin – recommended in all patients who have MS and atrial fibrillation
- diuretics – used to treat the pulmonary and peripheral oedema.

Mitral valvuloplasty

Mitral valvuloplasty involves the passage of a balloon across the mitral valve and its inflation, so stretching the stenosed valve. This procedure is carried out via a percutaneous route and only requires a local anaesthetic and light sedation. The following features make a patient unsuitable for this procedure:

- Marked mitral regurgitation
- A history of systemic emboli
- Calcified or thickened rigid mitral valve leaflets.

Surgical management

This is indicated in patients who have a mitral valve area of 1 cm² or less. Note that restenosis may occur after any valvuloplasty or valvotomy. In carefully selected patients this does not occur for many years; early restenosis within 5 years may occur in those who have thickened or rigid valves.

Open mitral valvotomy

Open mitral valvotomy is performed under general anaesthetic using a median sternotomy incision and requires cardiopulmonary bypass. It is used in patients who have already had a mitral valvuloplasty or who have mild mitral regurgitation.

Closed mitral valvotomy

This has now been superseded by mitral valvuloplasty. It does not require cardiopulmonary bypass; a curved incision is made under the left breast. It is worth knowing this because patients in finals examinations may have this scar.

Mitral valve replacement

This is used for calcified or very rigid valves unsuitable for valvuloplasty or valvotomy.

MITRAL REGURGITATION

The mitral valve may become incompetent for four reasons (Fig. 18.4):

1. Abnormal mitral valve annulus
2. Abnormal mitral valve leaflets
3. Abnormal chordae tendineae
4. Abnormal papillary muscle function.

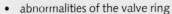

When considering the causes of regulation of any valve it is useful to divide the causes into:
- abnormalities of the valve ring
- abnormalities of the valve cusps and leaflets
- abnormalities of the supporting structures.

Pathophysiology

In mitral regurgitation (MR) the regurgitant jet of blood flows back into the left atrium and with time the left atrium dilates and accommodates the increased volume and pressure. There is, however, also increased backpressure in the pulmonary veins and as the MR worsens pulmonary hypertension develops, which may eventually cause RVF.

The left ventricle is dilated, because the blood entering from the left atrium with each beat is increased; over time this results in LVF. Therefore, severe, chronic MR if untreated, will result in biventricular failure. (Mitral stenosis differs because it does not cause LVF.)

Clinical features

These vary depending upon whether the MR is chronic or acute:

- Chronic mitral regurgitation develops slowly so allowing the heart to compensate and usually presents with a history of fatigue and dyspnoea.
- Acute MR presents with severe dyspnoea due to pulmonary oedema. The left atrium has not had time to dilate to accommodate the increased volume due to regurgitation of blood back through the mitral valve. The pressure increase is, therefore, transmitted directly to the pulmonary veins, resulting in pulmonary oedema.

Acute MR can be rapidly fatal and needs to be looked for in patients following myocardial infarction (MI) (papillary muscle rupture occurs at days 4–7 after MI, but papillary muscle dysfunction may occur earlier) and in patients who have infective endocarditis.

Site of pathology	Pathology
Mitral annulus	Senile calcification Left ventricular dilatation and enlargement of the annulus Abscess formation during infective endocarditis
Mitral valve leaflets	Infective endocarditis Rheumatic fever Prolapsing (floppy) mitral valve Congenital malformation Connective tissue disorders – Marfan syndrome, Ehlers–Danlos syndrome, osteogenesis imperfecta, pseudoxanthoma elasticum
Chordae tendinae	Idiopathic rupture Myxomatous degeneration Infective endocarditis Connective tissue disorders
Papillary muscle	Myocardial infarction Infiltration – sarcoid, amyloid Myocarditis

Fig. 18.4 Causes of mitral regurgitation

Examination

Features that may be seen are illustrated in Fig. 18.5 and include the following:

- Atrial fibrillation – an irregularly irregular pulse is common, especially in patients who have chronic MR and a dilated left atrium.
- Jugular venous pressure may be elevated – if the patient has developed pulmonary hypertension and right-heart failure, or fluid retention.
- The apex is displaced downward and laterally as the left ventricle dilates – eventually LVF may result. (Note that in MS the apex is not displaced because the left ventricle is protected by the stenosed mitral valve.)
- The murmur of MR is pansystolic and best heard at the apex – the murmur radiates to the axilla. Note that the loudness of the murmur is not an indicator of the severity of the MR.
- Signs of congestive cardiac failure – i.e. third heart sound, bilateral basal inspiratory crepitations, ascites and peripheral oedema.
- P_2 may be loud and there may be a right ventricular heave – if pulmonary hypertension has developed.

Floppy mitral valve

This is also known as mitral valve prolapse. Factors to consider are:

- this is a common disorder affecting approximately 4% of the population and more females than males
- the mitral valve may merely prolapse minimally into the left atrium or cause varying degrees of MR
- most cases are idiopathic, but floppy mitral valve is seen with greater frequency in certain conditions (e.g. Marfan syndrome and other connective tissue disorders)
- most patients are asymptomatic, the disorder being diagnosed at routine medical examination. Some patients present with fatigue, atypical chest pain and palpitations.
- examination reveals a mid-systolic click at the apex. This may or may not be followed by a systolic murmur of mitral regurgitation.
- prophylaxis against infective endocarditis is only indicated in those patients who have MR
- most patients require no further treatment other than reassurance.

Investigations

The following investigations may aid diagnosis.

Electrocardiography

There may be atrial fibrillation and left-ventricular hypertrophy.

Fig. 18.5 Clinical findings in patients who have mitral regurgitation. A_2, aortic component of second heart sound; AF, atrial fibrillation; CCF, congestive cardiac failure; P_2, pulmonary component of second heart sound.

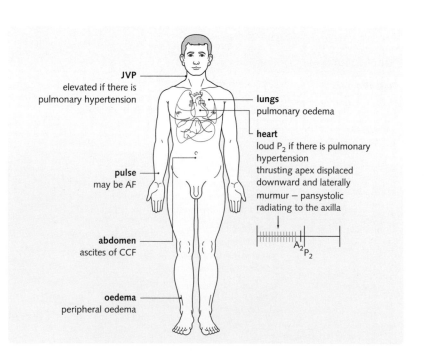

Chest radiography

An enlarged left ventricle may be seen as an increase in the cardiothoracic ratio. The mitral valve may be calcified and, therefore, visible.

Echocardiography

The mitral valve can be clearly seen and the regurgitant jet visualized. The left atrial size and left-ventricular size and function can be assessed. Suitability for mitral valve repair is better evaluated with TOE.

Cardiac catheterization

Most patients have minimal MR on echocardiography and do not require catheterization. This is performed to assess the severity of the MR and to exclude other valve lesions and coronary artery disease.

Management

Medical management

This may consist of diuretics and ACE inhibitors to treat the congestive cardiac failure.

Surgical management

Patients are considered for surgery if the MR is severe at echocardiography and cardiac catheterization. It is important to act before irreversible left ventricular damage and severe pulmonary hypertension have occurred.

Mitral valve repair

This may take the form of mitral annuloplasty, repair of a ruptured chorda or repair of a mitral valve leaflet. These procedures are performed on patients who have mobile non-calcified and non-thickened valves.

Mitral valve replacement

This is performed if mitral valve repair is not possible. Both repair and replacement of the mitral valve require a median sternotomy incision and cardiopulmonary bypass.

AORTIC STENOSIS

The most common form of aortic stenosis (AS) is valvular AS; however, aortic stenosis may also occur at the sub- or supravalvular level (Fig. 18.6).

Pathophysiology

The left-ventricular outflow obstruction results in an increased left-ventricular pressure. The left-ventricle undergoes hypertrophy and more vigorous and prolonged contraction to overcome the obstruction and maintain an adequate cardiac output. Myocardial oxygen demand is increased and, because systole is prolonged, diastole is shortened and, therefore, myocardial blood supply from the coronary arteries is reduced (coronary artery flow occurs during diastole; see *Crash course: cardiovascular system*).

Fig. 18.6 Causes of aortic stenosis

Type of AS	Cause
Valvular AS	Congenital most common, males > females (deformed valve can be uni-, bi-, or tricuspid)
	Senile calcification
	Rheumatic fever
	Severe atherosclerosis
Subvalvular AS	Fibromuscular ring
	HOCM
Supravalvular AS	Associated with hypercalcaemia in Williams syndrome, a syndrome associated with elfin facies, mental retardation, strabismus, hypervitaminosis D and hypercalcaemia; the inheritance is autosomal dominant

HOCM, hypertrophic obstructive cardiomyopathy.

Fig. 18.9 Clinical findings in patients who have aortic regurgitation. A$_2$, aortic component of second heart sound; S$_1$, first heart sound; S$_2$, second heart sound.

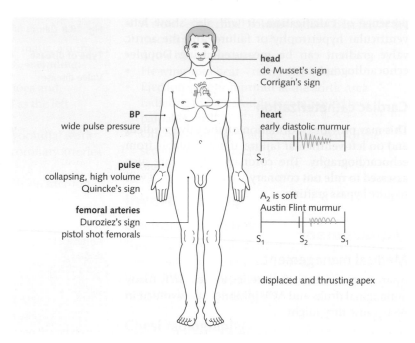

- a wide pulse pressure on measuring blood pressure
- downward and laterally displaced apex, which has a thrusting nature
- murmur best heard at the left lower sternal edge with the patient sitting forward and in full expiration – it is a soft high-pitched early diastolic murmur, which is sometimes difficult to hear, so be sure to listen for it properly with a diaphragm
- increased flow across the aortic valve may produce an ejection systolic murmur
- may be signs of left-ventricular or congestive failure
- other signs include de Musset's sign (head bobbing with each beat), Corrigan's sign (prominent pulsation in the neck), Quincke's sign (visible capillary pulsation in the nailbed), pistol shot femoral pulses (an audible femoral sound) and Duroziez's sign (another audible murmur over the femoral arteries – a to-and-fro sound)
- the Austin Flint murmur – heard when the regurgitant jet causes vibration of the anterior mitral valve leaflet. The murmur is similar to that of MS, but with no opening snap.

Investigations

Electrocardiography

This shows left-ventricular hypertrophy.

Chest radiography

The left ventricle may be enlarged and there may be pulmonary oedema.

Echocardiography

The structure of the aortic valve and the size of the regurgitant jet may be seen. Aortic root size and left-ventricular function can be assessed.

Cardiac catheterization

This enables assessment of aortic root size, severity of aortic regurgitation, left-ventricular function and co-existent coronary artery disease.

Management

Medical management

The use of diuretics and ACE inhibitors is valuable to treat cardiac failure in these patients. It is, however, important to make the diagnosis and surgically treat this condition before the left ventricle dilates and fails.

Surgical management

Aortic valve replacement is considered if the patient is symptomatic or if there are signs of progressive left-ventricular dilatation. The aortic root may also need to be replaced if it is grossly dilated.

Once a valve lesion has been diagnosed it is useful to be able to comment on its severity. This is judged by clinical, echocardiographic and angiographic means in most cases (Fig. 18.10).

TRICUSPID REGURGITATION

Causes

Most cases of tricuspid regurgitation (TR) are due to dilatation of the tricuspid annulus resulting from dilatation of the right ventricle. This may be due to any cause of RVF or pulmonary hypertension.

Occasionally, the tricuspid valve is affected by infective endocarditis (usually in intravenous drug abusers). Rarer causes include congenital malformations and the carcinoid syndrome.

Ebstein's anomaly

This congenital malformation is caused by downward displacement of the tricuspid valve into the body of the right ventricle. The valve is regurgitant and malformed. The condition is associated with other structural cardiac abnormalities and there is a high incidence of both supraventricular and ventricular tachyarrhythmias.

Clinical features

The symptoms and signs are due to the backpressure effects of the regurgitant jet into the right atrium, which are transmitted to the venous system causing a prominent v wave in the jugular venous waveform (Fig. 18.11).

Fatigue and discomfort, owing to ascites or hepatic congestion, are the commonest features. Patients usually present with symptoms of the disease causing the underlying RVF; the TR is often an incidental finding.

Management

The mainstay of management is medical with diuretics and angiotensin-converting enzyme inhibitors to treat the RVF and fluid overload. Tricuspid valve replacement is considered in very severe cases.

OTHER VALVE LESIONS

These are summarized in Fig. 18.12.

Fig. 18.10 Features indicating severity of valve disease

Valve disease	Features
MS	Proximity of opening snap to second heart sound and duration of murmur Valve area assessed on echocardiography Evidence of pulmonary hypertension on echocardiography and cardiac catheterization
MR	Symptoms and signs of pulmonary oedema Size of regurgitant jet and poor left ventricular function on echocardiography Evidence of pulmonary hypertension on echocardiography and cardiac catheterization
AS	Presence of symptoms Low-volume pulse and BP, obscured or absent aortic second sound Severity of aortic gradient and poor left ventricular function on echocardiography or cardiac catheterization
AR	Signs of LVF Left ventricular function and size of regurgitant jet on echocardiography or cardiac catheterization

AS, aortic stenosis; AR, aortic regurgitation; BP, blood pressure; LVF, left ventricular failure; MS, mitral stenosis; MR, mitral regurgitation.

Infective endocarditis

Objectives

By the end of this chapter you should:

- be able to list the cardiac conditions that predispose to endocarditis
- be aware of the complications of infective endocarditis
- be able to recognize the clinical signs of endocarditis
- understand the principles of antibiotic therapy in infective endocarditis
- be able to define the indications for surgery in infective endocarditis.

DEFINITION OF INFECTIVE ENDOCARDITIS

Infective endocarditis describes the condition where there is infection of the endothelial surface of the heart by a microorganism. Heart valves are most commonly affected, but any area causing a high-pressure jet through a narrow orifice may be involved (e.g. ventricular septal defect).

EPIDEMIOLOGY OF INFECTIVE ENDOCARDITIS

Infective endocarditis is an evolving disease. Traditionally, the main predisposing condition was rheumatic fever; however, the incidence of rheumatic fever in developed countries has dropped significantly because of improved social conditions and antibiotic therapy. Now, in developed countries different groups of patients are presenting with infective endocarditis for the following reasons:

- Increased number of prosthetic valve insertions
- Increased number of patients who have congenital heart disease surviving to adulthood
- Increasing elderly population
- Increasing intravenous drug abuse
- Antibiotic resistance.

With this change in the population affected by infective endocarditis, the organisms are also changing; for example, coagulase-negative staphylococci, which used to be uncommon, are now the most common organisms seen on prosthetic valves (Fig. 19.1).

People with the conditions listed in Fig. 19.2 should be advised about the importance of antibiotic prophylaxis before certain procedures to prevent infective endocarditis. These procedures are:

- any dental work
- any operation
- any instrumentation of the urinary tract
- any transrectal procedure (e.g. prostatic biopsy or colonoscopy with biopsy).

Oesophagogastroduodenoscopy is not thought to require antibiotic prophylaxis.

PATHOPHYSIOLOGY OF INFECTIVE ENDOCARDITIS

The development of endocarditis depends on a number of factors:

- Presence of anatomical abnormalities in the heart surface
- Haemodynamic abnormalities within the heart
- Host immune response
- Virulence of the organism
- Presence of bacteraemia.

Transient bacteraemia is a common occurrence, but infective endocarditis is rare so a healthy individual degree of valvular incompetence. The murmur of mitral regurgitation may become louder as the regurgitation gets worse. The murmur of aortic regurgitation also gets louder.

- Splenomegaly – a common finding especially if the history is long.
- Clubbing – develops after a few weeks of infective endocarditis. Other causes of clubbing include cyanotic congenital heart disease, suppurative lung disease, squamous cell carcinoma of the lung and inflammatory bowel disease.
- Splinter haemorrhages – more than four is pathological (remember that the most common cause of these is trauma).
- Osler's nodes and Janeway lesions – represent peripheral emboli (possibly septic).
- Roth's spots – retinal haemorrhages with a pale centre.
- Evidence of congestive cardiac failure.
- Microscopic haematuria on urine dipstick – always ask to dipstick the urine if you suspect infective endocarditis. This is a very sensitive test and easily carried out.
- Also peripheral emboli, features of a cerebrovascular event, inflamed joints.

INVESTIGATION OF A PATIENT WHO HAS INFECTIVE ENDOCARDITIS

Blood tests

Blood cultures

These are the most important investigations. Note the plural has been used because at least three sets of cultures must be performed. If possible, at least three sets should be taken at least 1 h apart *before* commencing antibiotic therapy. (If the patient is very ill and there is a high index of suspicion of infective endocarditis, it is appropriate to start antibiotics after the first set has been obtained, otherwise it is preferable to isolate the causative organism first.)

Positive blood cultures are usually obtained in at least 95% cases of bacterial endocarditis if taken before antibiotic therapy. This allows therapy to be specifically directed according to the sensitivity of the organism.

When taking blood cultures it is important to maintain a good aseptic technique to minimize the risk of contaminating the samples. Clean the skin with iodine-containing skin wash (or the equivalent if the patient has iodine allergy). Take the blood and then inject it into the culture bottles, using new needles.

Full blood count

Anaemia of chronic disease is common in patients who have less acute presentations. Other findings can include:

- leucocytosis – may be seen as a sign of inflammation (usually a neutrophilia)
- thrombocytopenia – may be an indication of disseminated intravascular coagulopathy
- thrombophilia – may be seen as part of the acute phase response.

Erythrocyte sedimentation rate and C-reactive protein

These are elevated as signs of inflammation. They are valuable markers of disease activity and repeated measurements every few days provide information on the patient's response to treatment.

Renal function

This may be impaired due to infarction or immune complex-mediated glomerulonephritis. This also needs repeating every few days during treatment as both aminoglycoside antibiotics and disease progression may cause renal impairment.

Liver function tests

These may be deranged due to septic microemboli.

Urinanalysis

As well as the bedside urine dipstick, formal urine microscopy should be performed to look for casts as seen in glomerulonephritis.

Chest radiography

This may be clear or may show signs of pulmonary oedema.

Echocardiography

Transthoracic echocardiography will reveal any valve incompetence and may also identify vegetations on the valve. This test is not very sensitive and cannot be used to exclude small vegetations.

Transoesophageal echocardiography is over 90% sensitive in diagnosing vegetations.

Remember that echocardiography is not a diagnostic test in infective endocarditis. It may help confirm the diagnosis and give information about the severity of the valve damage, but blood cultures are the only specific diagnostic test of infective endocarditis.

The diagnosis of infective endocarditis relies on the Duke criteria, requiring two major criteria, or one major plus three minor, or five minor.

Major criteria include:

- positive blood cultures (two or more with the same organism 12 h apart)
- evidence of endocardial involvement, e.g. vegetations on echocardiography, abscess or new valvar regurgitation

Minor criteria are:

- fever >38°C
- vascular phenomena, e.g. arterial emboli, mycotic aneurysm, septic pulmonary infarcts and Janeway lesions
- immunological phenomena, e.g. glomerulo-nephritis, Roth spots or Osler's nodes
- predisposition to endocarditis
- additional microbiological evidence not meeting major criteria.

MANAGEMENT OF INFECTIVE ENDOCARDITIS

There are two main aims in the management of infective endocarditis:

1. To treat the infection effectively with appropriate antibiotics with the minimum of drug-related complications
2. To diagnose and treat complications of the endocarditis (i.e. congestive cardiac failure, severe valve incompetence, peripheral abscesses, renal failure, etc.).

Antibiotic therapy

If infective endocarditis is suspected and the patient is unwell, antibiotic therapy is started as soon as the blood cultures have been taken (Fig. 19.5). The choice of agent can then be modified once the organism is known. Intravenous therapy is used initially in all cases. This may be via the central or peripheral route. It is vital that the intravenous access sites are changed regularly to prevent infection (peripheral lines every 3 days, non-tunnelled central lines every 5–7 days). The sites should be inspected regularly and the line removed immediately if there is evidence of local infection.

Fig. 19.5 Suggested antibiotic regimens

Organism	Suggested agents	Adverse effects
Streptococcus viridans	Benzylpenicillin 2.4 g IV 4-hourly (usually a 6-week course) and gentamicin	Allergic reactions; penicillin – interstitial nephritis; gentamicin – eighth cranial nerve and renal toxicity
Staphylococcus epidermidis	Benzylpenicillin or flucloxacillin IV; fucidic acid may be added	Fucidic acid – vomiting and hepatotoxicity
Staphylococcus aureus	Flucloxacillin and fucidic acid IV; gentamicin may also be useful initially. Cover for MRSA with vancomycin or teicoplanin until sensitivities known	
Gram-negative organisms	Ampicillin and gentamicin IV (dose according to levels)	gentamicin – eighth cranial nerve and renal toxicity
Yeasts	Flucytosine or amphotericin B	Flucytosine – marrow depression and hepatic failure; amphotericin – renal failure

IV, intravenously.

Objectives

By the end of this chapter you should:

- know the criteria for the diagnosis of hypertension
- be able to list the causes of secondary hypertension
- be able to outline the investigations you would request in a patient with hypertension and the reasons for each
- be able to describe the non-pharmacological measures to treat hypertension
- be able to list the major drug classes used in treatment of hypertension and outline their adverse effects
- be able to recognize phaeochromocytoma as a cause of hypertension and understand the investigations and management steps involved.

Hypertension is a major risk factor for cerebrovascular disease, myocardial infarction (MI), cardiac failure, peripheral vascular disease and renal failure. To reduce the risk of these it is important to diagnose and adequately treat hypertensive patients.

Whenever trying to learn a list of causes like the one in Fig. 20.1, most of your effort should be spent learning the main headings in the first column. Once you know these you will find your memory is triggered and you'll be able to recall at least two conditions for each category.

DEFINITION OF HYPERTENSION

Normal blood pressure increases with age and varies throughout the day according to factors such as stress and exertion. There is also an underlying diurnal variation, with the lowest blood pressure occurring at around 4 a.m.

The definition of hypertension, therefore, is that level of blood pressure associated with an increased risk of complications. This equates to a level above 140/90 mmHg in adults.

CLINICAL FEATURES OF HYPERTENSION

These are described in Chapter 7 and will not be repeated word for word here. The following is a summary of the clinical features of hypertension.

History

Most patients are entirely asymptomatic, but the presenting complaint may be headache, dizziness, fainting or visual disturbance.

CAUSES OF HYPERTENSION

Over 95% cases of hypertension are idiopathic and this is termed essential hypertension.

Secondary causes of hypertension, although rare, are important to exclude because they may be curable (Fig. 20.1).

There is no correlation between symptoms and severity of hypertension in the vast majority of patients.

hypertension the following screening tests should exclude most causative conditions:

- 24-h urine protein and creatinine clearance to exclude marked renal pathology
- 24-h urine catecholamines or vanillylmandelic acid (VMA) and 5-hydroxy indole acetic acid (5HIAA) to exclude phaeochromocytoma and carcinoid syndrome, respectively (three sets of urinary catecholamines should be tested)
- 24-h urine cortisol excretion and dexamethasone suppression test to exclude Cushing's syndrome
- Renal ultrasound to reveal any overt structural abnormality (e.g. phaeochromocytoma, small kidney or polycystic kidneys).
- Renal perfusion scan (diethylenetriamine pentaacetic acid, DTPA) with and without angiotensin-converting enzyme (ACE) inhibition to exclude renal artery stenosis. The kidney in renal artery stenosis depends heavily upon increased levels of angiotensin II to provide adequate blood pressure for renal perfusion. This is abruptly stopped by the administration of an ACE inhibitor and the reduction in renal blood flow that results can be detected by the scan. If this test is positive then renal angiography or MRA is the gold standard investigation to confirm the diagnosis.

MANAGEMENT OF HYPERTENSION

Importance of treating hypertension

Hypertension is a common disorder that, if left untreated, damages a number of systems. Complications of hypertension include:

- cardiac failure
- renal failure
- stroke
- ischaemic heart disease
- peripheral vascular disease.

This end-organ damage can largely be prevented by adequate blood pressure control.

However, hypertension is difficult to diagnose because patients are often asymptomatic. Treatment is, therefore, difficult because patients are less likely to comply with drug regimens or follow-up visits to their doctor.

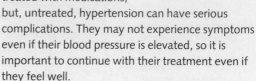

Explain to patients that hypertension can be well treated with medications, but, untreated, hypertension can have serious complications. They may not experience symptoms even if their blood pressure is elevated, so it is important to continue with their treatment even if they feel well.

Non-pharmacological management

This is important because in patients who have mild hypertension it may result in a moderate decrease in blood pressure of 11/8 mmHg and this may be sufficient to avoid the need for drug therapy. The following non-pharmacological treatments are recognized:

- Weight loss
- Reduction in alcohol consumption (currently, the maximum recommended weekly intakes are 28 units for men and 21 units for women)
- Reduction in salt intake
- Regular exercise.

All other risk factors for ischaemic heart disease should be sought and treated in these patients as a matter of routine.

Pharmacological management

There are many effective agents (Fig. 20.4). The main categories are as follows:

- Diuretics
- Antiadrenergic agents – β-blockers (β-adrenoceptor antagonists), α-blockers (α-adrenoceptor antagonists) and centrally acting agents
- Calcium channel blockers.

The use of β-blockers alone for phaeochromocytoma can result in severe hypertension due to the unopposed action of noradrenaline on the α-receptors.

- ACE inhibitors and angiotensin II receptor blockers
- Vasodilators.

Fig. 20.4 Overview of drugs used to treat hypertension

Class of drug	Examples	Indications	Precautions/ Contraindications	Adverse effects
Diuretics	Thiazides (e.g. bendroflumethiazide (bendrofluazide)) loop diuretics (e.g. furosemide (frusemide))	Mild hypertension or in conjunction with other agents for more severe hypertension	Thiazides exacerbate diabetes mellitus; all diuretics should be avoided in patients who have gout if possible	Hypokalaemia, dehydration, exacerbation of renal impairment, gout
Antiadrenergic agents	β-blockers (e.g. atenolol, propranolol, metoprolol)	Moderate to severe hypertension (note that they are antianginal)	Asthma, cardiac failure, severe peripheral vascular disease	Postural hypotension, bronchospasm, fatigue, impotence, cold extremities
	α-blockers (e.g. prazosin, doxazosin)	Moderate to severe hypertension	Postural hypotension	
	Centrally acting agents (e.g. methyldopa)	Moderate hypertension (safe during pregnancy)	Postural hypotension, galactorrhoea, gynaecomastia, haemolytic anaemia	
Calcium channel blockers	Nifedipine, amlodipine,	Moderate hypertension*	Cardiac failure, heart block (second or third degree) – these are contraindications mainly for verapamil and diltiazem	Postural hypotension, headache, flushing, ankle oedema
ACE inhibitors	Captopril, enalapril, lisinopril	Moderate to severe hypertension, especially with cardiac failure	Renal artery stenosis, pregnancy	Postural hypotension, dry cough, loss of taste, renal failure, hyperkalaemia
Angiotensin-II receptor blockers	Losartan, valsartan	Moderate to severe hypertension, especially with cardiac failure	Renal artery stenosis, pregnancy	Postural hypotension, renal failure, hyperkalaemia
Vasodilators	Hydralazine	Moderate to severe hypertension	SLE	Postural hypotension, headache, lupus-like syndrome
	Sodium nitroprusside (as an intravenous infusion)	Malignant hypertension		Weakness, cyanide toxicity if drug not protected from light

ACE, angiotensin-converting enzyme; SLE, systemic lupus erythematosus. *Diltiazem and verapamil are less commonly used for hypertension because they have a more pronounced action on heart muscle and conductive tissue, respectively. Diltiazem is used predominantly for angina; verapamil for its antiarrythmic effects.

173

These agents may be used alone or in combination to achieve good blood-pressure control. Remember that patient compliance is likely to be better if:

- the disease and its complications have been fully explained
- the treatment options have been discussed with the patient
- the drugs used have been explained and common side effects discussed
- once-daily preparations are used
- polypharmacy is avoided (i.e. the drug regimen is kept as simple as possible by using a higher dose of a single agent before adding another drug).

Recommended treatment of hypertension

The 2006 NICE/British Hypertension Society guidelines for the treatment of hypertension suggest:

- using non-pharmacological measures in all hypertensive and borderline hypertensive people
- initiating antihypertensive drug treatment in people with sustained systolic blood pressure =160 mmHg or sustained diastolic pressure =100 mmHg
- considering treatment in people with sustained systolic blood pressure between 140 and 159 mmHg or sustained diastolic blood pressure between 90 and 99 mmHg in the presence of target organ damage, cardiovascular disease or diabetes
- optimal blood pressure treatment targets are systolic blood pressure <140 mmHg and diastolic blood pressure <85 mmHg (or <130/80 mmHg in diabetics).

The choice of drug(s) to treat newly diagnosed hypertension is suggested in the NICE/BHS guidelines (www.nice.org.uk/CG034).

These guidelines are changing constantly (most up-to-date guidelines please refer to www.bhsoc.org) and clinical practice varies from hospital to hospital.

Follow-up of patients who have hypertension

This is every bit as important as the initial treatment. Patients should be seen on a 1- or 2-monthly basis until the blood pressure is less than 140/90 mmHg, and then on a yearly basis. The yearly follow-up should involve:

- examination to look for evidence of end-organ damage – especially cardiovascular system and retinas

- urine dipstick
- ECG
- blood tests for urea, creatinine and electrolytes – these may be deranged due to renal damage secondary to hypertension or to the drug therapy or both
- echocardiography if the patient had left-ventricular hypertrophy at diagnosis – it is appropriate to repeat the echocardiography until the hypertrophy has resolved
- a screen of risk factors for ischaemic heart disease (i.e. blood lipid profile and blood glucose) and lifestyle advice if necessary.

PHAEOCHROMOCYTOMA

Phaeochromocytoma is a rare tumour of the chromaffin cells – 90% occur within the adrenal medulla and 10% are extramedullary; 10% are malignant and 10% are bilateral.

Clinical features

Paroxysmal catecholamine secretion results in a variety of signs and symptoms including:

- hypertension
- headaches
- sweating attacks
- postural hypotension
- acute pulmonary oedema.

These symptoms are characteristically paroxysmal, although patients might have persistent hypertension.

Investigations

Investigations include:

- ECG-ST elevation or T wave inversion may be seen transiently
- echocardiography – shows left-ventricular hypertrophy or dilated cardiomyopathy
- 24-h urinary catecholamines or VMA – these are raised (at least three measurements should be taken because of the intermittent nature of the catecholamine excretion)
- computed tomography of the adrenals or meta-iodobenzylguanidine (MIBG) scan if the tumour is extra-adrenal
- selective venous sampling.

Management

Careful blood pressure control is vital before any invasive procedure as follows:

- Initially, α-blocker is used (phenoxybenzamine, an irreversible α-blocker, is commonly used)
- β-Blockade may then be added if required – the use of β-blockers alone may result in severe hypertension due to the unopposed action of noradrenaline on the α-receptors.

The tumour is then removed surgically.

Further reading

NICE/BHS guidelines www.nice.org.uk/CG034

ESC Guidelines Committee 2003 European Society of Cardiology guidelines for the management of arterial hypertension. *Journal of Hypertension* **21**: 1011–53

Padwal R, Straus S E, McAlister F A 2001 Evidence based management of hypertension: Cardiovascular risk factors and their effects on the decision to treat hypertension: evidence based review. *BMJ* **322**: 977–80

Objectives

By the end of this chapter you should:

- be able to list the congenital heart diseases that are associated with cyanosis
- be able to outline the different types of atrial septal defect
- be able to recognize the clinical signs of a ventricular septal defect
- be able to describe the pathophysiological process that occurs if a significant intracardiac shunt is untreated
- be able to define the four main features of tetralogy of Fallot.

DEFINITION OF CONGENITAL HEART DISEASE

Congenital heart disease refers to cardiac lesions present from birth.

CAUSES OF CONGENITAL HEART DISEASE

Many factors both genetic and environmental affect cardiac development in the uterus; therefore, not surprisingly, no one cause can explain all cases (Fig. 21.1). These include:

- maternal rubella – in addition to cataracts, deafness and microcephaly, this can cause patent ductus arteriosus (PDA) and pulmonary stenosis
- fetal alcohol syndrome – associated with cardiac defects (as well as microcephaly, micrognathia, microphthalmia and growth retardation).
- maternal systemic lupus erythematosus – associated with fetal complete heart block (due to transplacental passage of anti-Ro antibodies).

There are many genetic associations with congenital heart disease, including:

- Trisomy 21 – endocardial cushion defects, atrial septal defect (ASD), ventricular septal defect (VSD) and Fallot's tetralogy
- Turner's syndrome (XO) – coarctation of the aorta
- Marfan syndrome – aortic dilatation and aortic and mitral regurgitation
- Kartagener's syndrome – dextrocardia.

COMPLICATIONS OF CONGENITAL HEART DISEASE

Before discussing individual lesions it is important to have a grasp of the significance of congenital heart disease. Lesions have effects depending upon their size and location. These include:

- cyanosis – defined as the presence of more than 5 g/dL of reduced haemoglobin in arterial blood. Central cyanosis can be caused by congenital heart disease due to shunting of venous blood straight into the arterial circulation bypassing the lungs. This type of cyanosis does not, therefore, respond to increasing the concentration of inspired oxygen

Notes on cyanosis:
- Central cyanosis is cyanosis of the tongue
- Peripheral cyanosis is cyanosis of the peripheries (lips, feet, hands, etc.)
- Cyanosis caused by pulmonary disease or cardiac failure improves on increasing inspired oxygen
- Cyanosis caused by a right-to-left shunt bypassing the lungs does not improve on increasing inspired oxygen.

- congestive cardiac failure – this occurs due to the inability of the heart to maintain sufficient tissue perfusion as a result of the cardiac lesion. This may occur in infancy (e.g. due to a large

Fig. 21.1 Cardiac malformations (in descending order of incidence)

Ventricular septal defect (VSD)
Atrial septal defect (ASD)
Patent ductus arteriosus (PDA)
Pulmonary stenosis – causes cyanosis if severe
Coarctation of the aorta
Aortic stenosis
Fallot's tetralogy – causes cyanosis
Transposition of the great arteries – causes cyanosis
Other causes of cyanotic congenital heart
disease – pulmonary atresia, hypoplastic left heart, severe
Ebstein's anomaly with ASD

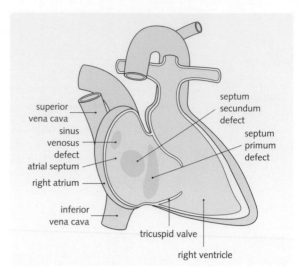

Fig. 21.2 Location of the three main types of atrial septal defect. The heart is viewed from the right side. The right atrial and ventricular walls have been omitted to reveal the septum.

VSD or transposition of the great arteries), or in adulthood in less severe conditions

- pulmonary hypertension – this develops over time as a result of an abnormal increase in pulmonary blood flow due to a left-to-right shunt (e.g. ASD, VSD, PDA). This increased flow results in changes to the pulmonary vessels with smooth muscle hypertrophy and obliterative changes. The pulmonary vascular resistance increases causing pulmonary hypertension. Eventually pulmonary pressure exceeds systemic pressure causing reversal of the shunt, and this results in a syndrome of cyanotic heart disease called Eisenmenger's syndrome.
- infective endocarditis – congenital heart disease may result in lesions prone to bacterial colonization. Appropriate antibiotic prophylaxis should be taken to prevent this.
- sudden death – this may be due to arrhythmias (more common in these disorders) or outflow tract obstruction as seen in aortic stenosis.

ATRIAL SEPTAL DEFECT

Although a common cause of congenital heart disease, atrial septal defect (ASD) is often not diagnosed early because it can be difficult to detect clinically.

There are three main types of ASD based on the location of the defect in the atrial septum (Fig. 21.2):

1. Septum primum (also called ostium primum ASD) – this defect lies adjacent to the atrioventricular valves and these are often also abnormal and incompetent.
2. Septum secundum (also called ostium secundum ASD) – the most common form of ASD, it is mid-septal in location.

3. Sinus venosus ASD – this lies high in the septum and may be associated with anomalous pulmonary venous drainage (where one of the pulmonary veins drains into the right atrium instead of the left).

Clinical features

The magnitude of the left-to-right shunt depends upon the size of the defect and also the relative pressures on the left and right sides of the heart.

History

In early life patients are usually asymptomatic. In adult life, however, symptoms of dyspnoea, fatigue and recurrent chest infections occur. As time goes by the increased pulmonary blood flow results in pulmonary hypertension and eventually reversal of the shunt and Eisenmenger's syndrome.

Examination

The findings on examination of a patient who has an ASD (Fig. 21.3) depend upon the following factors:

- Size of the ASD
- Presence or absence of pulmonary hypertension
- Presence of shunt reversal.

The second heart sound is widely split because closure of the pulmonary valve is delayed due to increased pulmonary blood flow. The splitting is fixed

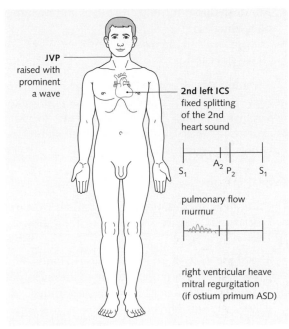

JVP
raised with
prominent
a wave

2nd left ICS
fixed splitting
of the 2nd
heart sound

S_1 A_2 P_2 S_1

pulmonary flow
murmur

right ventricular heave
mitral regurgitation
(if ostium primum ASD)

Fig. 21.3 Physical findings in all patients who have an atrial septal defect (ASD). If the ASD is large and there is pulmonary hypertension, check for loud P_2 at the second left intercostal space (ICS) and for a prominent right ventricular heave. If there is shunt reversal you will find clubbing, central cyanosis and signs of congestive cardiac failure (i.e. peripheral oedema, ascites and bilateral basal crepitations). A_2, aortic component of second heart sound; JVP, jugular venous pressure; P_2, pulmonary component of second heart sound; S_1, first heart sound.

in relation to respiration because the communication between the atria prevents the normal pressure differential between right and left sides that occurs during respiration. This is referred to as fixed splitting of the second heart sound.

The increased pulmonary blood flow causes a mid-systolic pulmonary flow murmur.

> Eisenmenger's syndrome can occur in any condition involving a left-to-right shunt. With worsening pulmonary hypertension the shunt eventually reverses (changes to right to left) causing blood to bypass the lungs and resulting in profound cyanosis that is not responsive to oxygen therapy. There is no treatment at this late stage.

If pulmonary hypertension has developed, there is reduction of the left-to-right shunt and the pulmonary flow murmur disappears; instead there is a loud pulmonary component to the second heart

sound because the increased pressure causes the pulmonary valve to slam shut.

If Eisenmenger's syndrome occurs the patient becomes centrally cyanosed and develops finger clubbing.

Investigation

Electrocardiography

Patients who have ostium secundum ASD usually have right axis deviation. Those who have an ostium primum defect have left axis deviation.

Chest radiography

The pulmonary artery appears dilated and its branches are prominent. The enlarged right atrium can be seen at the right heart border and the enlarged right ventricle causes rounding of the left heart border.

Echocardiography

The right side of the heart and the pulmonary artery are dilated. The ASD may be directly visualized and a jet of blood may be seen passing through it. Associated mitral or tricuspid valve incompetence may be seen.

Cardiac catheterization

This again reveals the ASD because the catheter can be passed across it. Serial oxygen saturation measurements are made at different levels from the superior vena cava through the atrium and the right ventricle into the pulmonary artery. At the level of the left-to-right shunt there will be a step-up increase of the oxygen saturation as blood from the left side enters the right. This measurement can be used to calculate the size of the shunt, which helps determine whether operative correction of the ASD is required.

Magnetic resonance imaging

This is increasingly used in assessment of patients with congenital heart disease. It offers excellent image quality and haemodynamic data and does not involve ionizing radiation.

Management

If there are signs of congestive cardiac failure, diuretics and angiotensin-converting enzyme inhibitors may be of benefit.

An ASD carries a risk of infective endocarditis so the appropriate prophylactic measures should be taken.

The primary aim in these patients is to diagnose the ASD early and evaluate its severity to be able to repair the defect before pulmonary hypertension occurs. Once the patient has developed pulmonary hypertension repair does not stop its deterioration.

All ASDs with pulmonary to systemic flow ratios exceeding 1.5:1 should be repaired.

Operative closure requires cardiopulmonary bypass and involves a median sternotomy scar.

A new technique has been developed where the ASD is closed percutaneously using a device with two deformable discs connected by a narrow waist. This is introduced via a cardiac catheter and involves only a venous puncture.

When asked about the management of any valve disease or congenital defect, many students forget that antibiotic prophylaxis is probably one of the most important aspects of management – so don't forget to put it high on your list of priorities.

VENTRICULAR SEPTAL DEFECT

This is the most common congenital cardiac abnormality.

The ventricular septum is made up of two main components:

1. The membranous septum – situated high in the septum and relatively small. This is the most common site for a VSD.
2. The muscular septum – this is lower and defects here may be multiple.

Clinical features

History

In the neonate, a small VSD will be asymptomatic but a large VSD will result in the development of left-ventricular failure. This occurs because in the neonate pulmonary pressures are very high and a right-to-left shunt occurs via the VSD; if this is very large the left ventricle cannot cope and fails. The signs of LVF in a neonate are as follows:

- Failure to thrive, feeding difficulties and sweating on feeding
- Tachypnoea and intercostal recession
- Hepatomegaly.

The adult who has a VSD may be asymptomatic or may present with dyspnoea due to pulmonary hypertension (which may develop over many years as a consequence of the left-to-right shunt) or Eisenmenger's syndrome.

Examination

The findings on examination of a patient who has a VSD (Fig. 21.4) vary according to the following criteria:

- Size of the VSD – a small VSD causes a loud pansystolic murmur that radiates to the apex and axilla. A very large VSD causes a less loud pansystolic murmur, but may be associated with signs of left ventricular and right ventricular hypertrophy.
- Presence or absence of pulmonary hypertension.
- Presence of shunt reversal.

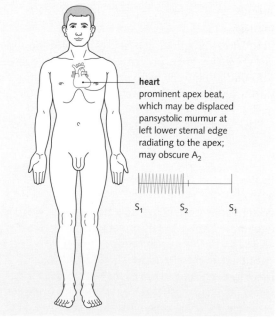

heart
prominent apex beat, which may be displaced pansystolic murmur at left lower sternal edge radiating to the apex; may obscure A_2

S_1 S_2 S_1

Fig. 21.4 Physical findings in all patients with a ventricular septal defect (VSD). If the VSD is large, the apex is displaced and pulmonary hypertension can develop. This results in a loud P_2 (pulmonary component of second heart sound) and right ventricular heave. Eisenmenger's syndrome might also develop, with clubbing, cyanosis and disappearance of the pansystolic murmur. A_2, aortic component of second heart sound; S_1, first heart sound; S_2, second heart sound.

Investigation

Chest radiography

This may show an enlarged left ventricle with prominent pulmonary vascular markings. Pulmonary oedema may be seen in infants.

Echocardiography

This will show the VSD and its size and location, and can help to evaluate the effects on cardiac function.

Magnetic resonance imaging

This can be used if further assessment is needed, or if the VSD is not well seen on echocardiography.

Management

Approximately 30% of cases close spontaneously, most of these by the time the child is 3 years of age. Some do not close until the child is 10 years old. Defects near the valve ring or near the outlet of the ventricle do not usually close.

Operative closure is the treatment of choice (if there is a significant left-to-right shunt) and is recommended for all lesions that have not undergone spontaneous closure. Some small lesions are managed conservatively; such a patient may be a case in finals and has a loud pansystolic murmur.

A VSD is a risk factor for infective endocarditis so the appropriate prophylactic measures should be taken.

PATENT DUCTUS ARTERIOSUS

In the fetus most of the output of the right ventricle bypasses the lungs via the ductus arteriosus. This vessel joins the pulmonary trunk (artery) to the descending aorta distal to the left subclavian artery (Fig. 21.5). The ductus arteriosus normally closes about 1 month after birth in full-term infants and takes longer to close in premature infants.

Clinical features

The factors that determine the nature of the clinical features are the same as in VSD and ASD (i.e. the size of the defect, the size of the shunt, the presence of pulmonary hypertension, and the development of Eisenmenger's syndrome).

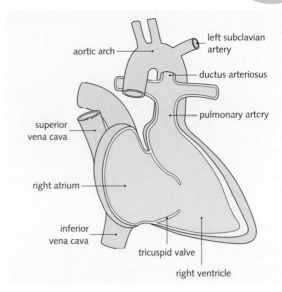

Fig. 21.5 Position of the ductus arteriosus.

A patent ductus arteriosus (PDA) is more likely in babies born at high altitude, probably due to the low atmospheric oxygen concentration. This lesion is also common in babies who have fetal rubella syndrome.

History

A small PDA is asymptomatic, but a large defect causes a large left-to-right shunt and may lead to left-ventricular failure (LVF) with pulmonary oedema causing failure to thrive and tachypnoea.

Adults who have undiagnosed PDA may develop pulmonary hypertension and present with dyspnoea.

Differential cyanosis occurs in adults with reversal of the shunt as the venous blood enters the systemic circulation below the subclavian arteries causing cyanosis and clubbing of the lower extremities whereas the arms remain pink.

Examination

The classic findings in a patient who has PDA (Fig. 21.6) are:

- collapsing high-volume pulses – this is due to the effect of the run-off of blood back down the ductus
- a loud continuous machinery murmur heard in the second left intercostal space
- a palpable thrill in the same place.

181

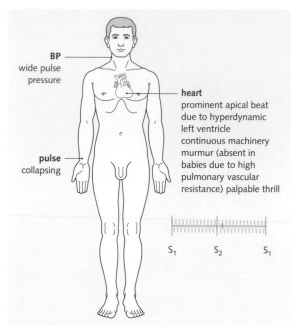

Fig. 21.6 Physical findings in all patients with patent ductus arteriosus (PDA). Patients with a large PDA have a loud pulmonary component of the second heart sound (P_2) due to pulmonary hypertension and the murmur is soft or absent. In those who have Eisenmenger's syndrome there is differential cyanosis and the toes are clubbed.

Management

The management of PDA involves two stages:

1. Pharmacological closure in neonates – indomethacin may induce closure if given early (by inhibiting prostacyclin production).
2. Operative closure of the PDA – this can be performed as an open procedure where the PDA is ligated or divided. Alternatively a percutaneous approach can be performed with introduction of an occluding device via a cardiac catheter. Antibiotic prophylaxis is required for all patients before operative correction because PDA is a risk factor for infective endocarditis.

COARCTATION OF THE AORTA

In this condition there is a congenital narrowing of the aorta, usually beyond the left subclavian artery.

There are two main types:

1. Infantile type – this presents soon after birth with heart failure.
2. Adult type – the obstruction develops more gradually and presents in early adulthood.

This type is associated with a high incidence of bicuspid aortic valve.

An adaptive response to the coarctation develops in those patients who do not present in infancy. This involves the development of collateral blood vessels, which divert blood from the proximal aorta to other peripheral arteries bypassing the obstruction. These collaterals are seen around the scapula as tortuous vessels that can sometimes be palpated and as prominent posterior intercostal arteries that cause rib notching visible on chest radiography. These collaterals take some years to develop and are rarely seen before 6 years of age.

Clinical features

History

Infants may present with failure to thrive and tachypnoea secondary to LVF. Alternatively coarctation may present as rapid severe cardiac failure with the infant in extremis.

Adults whose condition is not diagnosed in childhood may present with:

- hypertension diagnosed at routine medical testing
- symptoms of leg claudication
- left ventricular failure
- subarachnoid haemorrhage from associated berry aneurysm
- angina pectoris due to premature heart disease.

Examination

Careful examination of these patients is vital because the diagnosis must not be missed. The physical findings in patients who have coarctation of the aorta are shown in Fig. 21.7. Check for:

- blood pressure – it is always important to take blood pressure in both arms whenever performing the cardiovascular examination. Aortic dissection and coarctation where the obstruction is proximal to the left subclavian artery both cause a pressure differential between the arms. The blood pressure in the legs is also lower than in the arms
- radiofemoral delay and weak leg pulses – it is important to always look for radiofemoral delay because it is diagnostic of this condition
- a heaving displaced apex beat due to left-ventricular hytertrophy

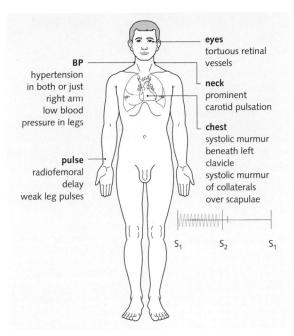

BP
hypertension
in both or just
right arm
low blood
pressure in legs

eyes
tortuous retinal
vessels

neck
prominent
carotid pulsation

chest
systolic murmur
beneath left
clavicle
systolic murmur
of collaterals
over scapulae

pulse
radiofemoral
delay
weak leg pulses

S_1 S_2 S_1

Fig. 21.7 Physical findings in patients with coarctation of the aorta. If the coarctation is severe there is a continuous murmur beneath the left clavicle and signs of left-ventricular failure (bilateral basal crepitations and audible third heart sound).

- murmurs – the coarctation may cause a systolic murmur (or a continuous murmur if the narrowing is very tight). This is located below the left clavicle. The collaterals cause an ejection systolic murmur that can be heard over the scapulae. There may be a murmur associated with a bicuspid aortic valve, which is ejection systolic in nature and is located over the aortic area.

Investigation

Electrocardiography

This reveals left ventricular hypertrophy and often right bundle branch block.

Chest radiography

Rib notching might be seen in children over 6 years of age. (Because the first and second intercostal arteries arise from the vertebral arteries there is no rib notching on these ribs.) The aortic knuckle is absent and a double knuckle is seen (made up of the dilated subclavian artery above and the poststenotic dilatation of the aorta below).

Echocardiography

The coarctation and any associated lesion may be visualized, but imaging the thoracic aorta can be difficult. Coarctation is associated with a number of other congenital abnormalities (e.g. bicuspid aortic valve, transposition of the great arteries, septum primum ASD and mitral valve disease).

Cardiac catheterization

This localizes the coarctation accurately and also provides more information on associated lesions.

Magnetic resonance imaging

This provides very good three-dimensional reconstruction of the coarctation and is a useful tool prior to treatment in order to correct the coarctation.

Management

The most popular first-line treatment is an operation to relieve the obstruction. Without correction the prognosis is extremely poor and most patients die by 40 years of age. Balloon angioplasty has emerged as an alternative first-line treatment and avoids the need for sternotomy and cardiopulmonary bypass.

Coarctation may be complicated by infective endocarditis so antibiotic prophylaxis should be used.

OTHER LESIONS IN CONGENITAL HEART DISEASE

The conditions discussed above are those most likely to be seen in the examination situation. There are, however, a number of less common congenital cardiac abnormalities and these are discussed in Fig. 21.8.

NOTES ON PULMONARY HYPERTENSION AND EISENMENGER'S SYNDROME

Pulmonary hypertension

This causes mild dyspnoea when the shunt is from left to right and severe dyspnoea with the progression of pulmonary hypertension. Signs on examination include:

Fig. 21.8 Uncommon causes of congenital cardiac abnormalities

Congenital cardiac defect	Anatomical abnormality	Clinical features	Treatment
Congenital aortic stenosis (acyanotic)	Stenosis may be valvular (most common), subvalvular, or supravalvular; note Williams syndrome – autosomal dominant condition with hypercalcaemia and supravalvular aortic stenosis	More common in males; child may be hypotensive, dyspnoeic and sweaty; increased incidence of angina and sudden death, especially on exertion; ejection systolic murmur heard in the second right ICS; may be signs of left ventricular strain (heaving apex) and failure (S_3, tachycardia and bilateral basal crackles)	Operative correction of the stenosis is the treatment of choice; in very small infants valvuloplasty is preferred in the first instance
Hypoplastic left heart (cyanotic)	Underdevelopment of all or part of the left side of the heart	Heart failure occurs in the first week of life; echocardiography is diagnostic	Surgical treatment is the only option and the mortality rate is extremely high
Pulmonary artery stenosis (cyanotic only if severe)	Stenosis at one or many points along the pulmonary arteries; associated with Fallot's tetralogy in some cases; complication of maternal rubella infection	If mild the patient may be asymptomatic with signs of RVH (i.e. left parasternal heave) and a pulmonary ejection systolic murmur; if severe blood flows from the right side to the left through the foramen ovale and the child is cyanosed and dyspnoeic	Diagnosis is confirmed by echocardiography; pulmonary angioplasty may provide a definitive cure; if there is a recurrence or the lesion is not suitable for pulmonary angioplasty the obstruction may be removed surgically
Tetralogy of Fallot (cyanotic)	Four components: (1) VSD; (2) pulmonary stenosis; (3) overriding aorta; (4) RVH – blood flow therefore passes from the right ventricle through the VSD and through the aorta, resulting in a right-to-left shunt	Most children present with cyanosis within the first year of life; patients may have 'spells' of intense cyanosis from time to time due to a sudden increase in the right to left shunt – these attacks can be terminated by squatting, which increases systemic resistance and therefore reduces the right-to-left shunt	Total surgical correction is the treatment of first choice; in very young infants who have severe pulmonary atresia a palliative operation to reduce the pulmonary obstruction usually provides relief and a definitive procedure can be carried out later, when the risk is lower
Complete transposition of the great arteries (cyanotic)	The aorta arises from the right ventricle and the pulmonary artery arises from the left ventricle – the two circulations are therefore parallel; death is rapid if there is no communication between them so it is also common to see an ASD, VSD or PDA in these infants	Early cardiac failure and cyanosis are the most common presenting features; symptoms are less severe in those infants who have a large communication between the two sides; diagnosis is made by echocardiography and cardiac catheterization	Medical treatment of cardiac failure and the use of prostaglandin E1 to prevent postnatal closure of the ductus can help; operative procedures to create a large ASD might also help in the short term; surgical correction of the transposition is the definitive treatment

ASD, atrial septal defect; ICS, intercostal space; PDA, patent ductus arteriosus; RVH, right ventricular hypertrophy; S_3, third heart sound; VSD, ventricular septal defect.

- dominant a wave in the jugular venous pulse
- palpable and loud pulmonary component of second heart sound
- ejection systolic murmur in pulmonary area due to increased flow
- right ventricular heave
- tricuspid regurgitation if the right ventricle dilates.

Echocardiography allows assessment of the pulmonary pressures. This is vital because the shunt should be corrected before significant pulmonary hypertension develops.

Eisenmenger's syndrome

This refers to the situation where a congenital cardiac abnormality initially causes acyanotic heart disease, but cyanotic heart disease develops as a consequence of raised pulmonary pressure and shunt reversal.

These clinical features are also seen in patients who have cyanotic congenital heart disease (i.e. where the lesion results in a right-to-left shunt from the outset). Cyanosis develops when the level of reduced haemoglobin is over 5 g/dL.

Dyspnoea is usually relatively mild considering the profound hypoxia these patients have (oxygen saturations of 50% are not uncommon).

Complications include:

- clubbing – develops in the fingers and toes
- polycythaemia and hyperviscosity – with resulting complications of stroke and venous thrombosis. Regular venesection or anticoagulation may be necessary

- cerebral abscesses – especially in children
- paradoxical emboli – emboli from venous thrombosis may pass across the shunt and give rise to systemic infarcts.

Female patients with congenital heart disease should be counselled regarding the potential risks of becoming pregnant and in appropriate cases be referred to a specialist at a stage when they are considering starting a family.

Further reading

Brickner M E, Hillis L D, Lange R A 2000 Congenital heart disease in adults. Part I *N Engl J Med* **342**: 256–63, Part II *N Engl J Med* **342**: 334–42

Gatzoulis M A, Webb G D (eds) 2003 Diagnosis and Management of Adult Congenital Heart Disease, 1st edn. Churchill Livingstone, Edinburgh

Task Force of the ESC 2003 Management of grown up congenital heart disease. *Eur Heart J* **24**(11): 1035–84

HISTORY, EXAMINATION AND COMMON INVESTIGATIONS

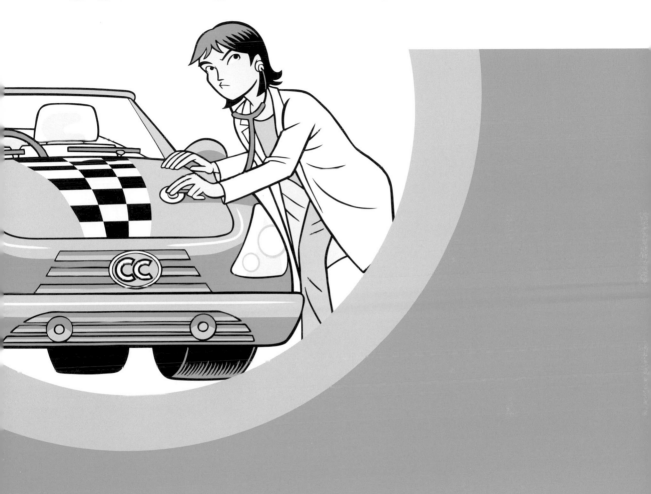

By the end of this chapter you should:

- be able to take a history from a patient – with specific relevance to symptoms that arise from cardiovascular disease
- understand the extra-cardiac symptoms that may arise from cardiovascular disease.

AIM OF HISTORY TAKING

The aim of history taking is to observe the following points:

- Highlight important symptoms and present them in a clear and logical manner
- Obtain information about the severity of the symptoms and, therefore, of the underlying disease
- Ask questions relevant to suspected diseases and so narrow the list of suspected differential diagnoses
- Evaluate to what extent the individual's lifestyle has been affected by or has contributed to the underlying disease.

PRESENTING COMPLAINT

The presenting complaint will usually be one of the following:

- Chest pain
- Dyspnoea
- Syncope or dizziness
- Ankle swelling
- Palpitations.

It may be an incidental finding of a murmur or hypertension as a reason for referral from a colleague.

The presenting complaint should be documented in a few words at the beginning of the clerking, and is followed by a more in-depth assessment, the history of the presenting complaint.

Chest pain

Ascertain the following points as you would for any type of pain:

- nature of the pain (e.g. sharp, dull, heavy, burning)
- site and radiation of the pain
- exacerbating and relieving factors
- duration of the problem – is it getting worse?
- associated features (Fig. 22.1).

Angina means 'choking'. Patients will often deny chest pain and will describe a squeezing or crushing sensation instead.

Dyspnoea

This is an uncomfortable awareness of one's breathing. Ascertain the following:

- Precipitating factors
- Duration of the problem – is it getting worse?
- Associated features, such as chest pain, palpitations, sweating, cough or haemoptysis (Fig. 22.2)
- Is the patient short of breath lying flat (orthopnoea) or do they wake up due to shortness of breath (paroxysmal nocturnal dyspnoea)?

Syncope

This is a loss of consciousness due to inadequate perfusion of the brain. The differential diagnosis is given in Fig. 22.3.

Paroxysmal nocturnal dyspnoea may be the first feature of pulmonary oedema. This occurs when fluid accumulates in the lungs when the patient lies flat during sleep. When awake, the respiratory centres are very sensitive and register oedema early with dyspnoea; during sleep sensory awareness is depressed, allowing pulmonary oedema to accumulate. The patient is, therefore, woken by a severe sensation of breathlessness, which is extremely frightening and is relieved by sitting or standing up.

Ask about the following:

- Speed of onset
- Precipitating events
- Nature of the recovery period.

Cardiac syncope often occurs with no warning and is associated with rapid and complete recovery. Be careful, therefore, because the patient will usually be well when you take the history despite having a potentially life-threatening condition.

Palpitations

Ask the following questions:

- Can you describe the palpitations (ask the patient to tap them out)?
- Are there any precipitating or relieving factors?
- How long do they last and how frequent are they?
- Are there any associated features (e.g. shortness of breath, chest pain or loss of consciousness; Fig. 22.4)?

Commonly used vagotonic manoeuvres include:

- valsalva manoeuvre (bearing down against a closed glottis)
- carotid sinus massage – remember only one side at a time and listen for carotid bruits beforehand
- painful stimuli (e.g. immersing the hands into iced water or ocular pressure)
- diving reflex (i.e. immersing the face in water).

Ankle swelling

Cardiac causes of ankle swelling include congestive cardiac failure (fluid retention caused by heart failure).

There are many causes of cardiac failure. Causes of left-heart failure include:

- ischaemic heart disease
- hypertension

Fig. 22.1 Features of different types of chest pain

Cause	Angina pectoris	Pericarditis	Pulmonary embolus or pneumonia	Oesophagitis or oesophageal spasm	Cervical spondylosis
Location	Retrosternal	Central or left-sided	Anywhere in chest	Epigastric or retrosternal	Central or lateral
Nature	Pressure or dull ache	Sharp	Sharp	Dull or burning	Aching or sharp
Radiation	Left arm, neck, or jaw	No	No	Neck	Arms
Exacerbating	Exertion, cold weather, stress	Recumbent position, deep inspiration	Deep inspiration, coughing	Recumbent position, presence or lack of food	Movement factors
Relieving features	Rest, GTN spray, oxygen mask	Sitting forward	Stopping breathing	Food or antacids, GTN spray	Weather, position in bed
Associated features	Shortness of breath, sweating, nausea, palpitations	Shortness of breath, sweating, palpitations, fever	Shortness of breath, haemoptysis, cough, fever	Sweating, nausea	Dizziness, pain in neck or shoulder

GTN, glyceryl trinitrate.

Fig. 22.2 Features of conditions causing dyspnoea

System involved	Disease	Features of dyspnoea
Cardiovascular	Pulmonary oedema	May be acute or chronic, exacerbated by exertion or lying flat (orthopnoea and PND), associated with sweating (and cough with pink frothy sputum)
	Ischaemic heart disease	Exacerbated by exertion or stress, relieved by rest, associated with sweating and angina
Respiratory	COPD	Chronic onset, exacerbated by exertion and respiratory infections, may be associated with cough and sputum, always associated with history of smoking
	Interstitial lung disease	Chronic onset, no real exacerbating or relieving factors, may have history of exposure to occupational dusts or allergens
	Pulmonary embolus	Acute onset, associated with pleuritic chest pain and haemoptysis
	Pneumothorax	Acute onset, pleuritic chest pain
	Pneumonia and neoplasms of the lung	Associated with pleuritic pain
Other	Pregnancy	Gradual progression due to splinting of diaphragm or anaemia
	Obesity	Gradual progression due to effort of moving and chest wall restriction
	Anaemia	History of blood loss, peptic ulcer, operations, etc

COPD, chronic obstructive pulmonary disease; PND, paroxysmal nocturnal dyspnoea.

- mitral and aortic valve disease
- cardiomyopathies
- congestive cardiac failure
- drug side effect, e.g. due to amlodipine (a calcium channel antagonist used to treat angina or hypertension).

Start with open questions and give the patient a chance to tell you in their own words what the problem is. Then probe with more specific questions about the nature of particular symptoms. Avoid putting words into the patient's mouth. For example, when asking about chest pain, use a neutral phrase such as: 'can you tell me what the discomfort is like?'

Causes of right-heart failure include.

- chronic lung disease (cor pulmonale)
- pulmonary embolism
- tricuspid and pulmonary valve disease

- mitral valve disease with pulmonary hypertension
- right ventricular infarct
- primary pulmonary hypertension.

From the above list it can be seen that a history encompassing all aspects of cardiac disease needs to be taken to identify the possible causes of ankle swelling.

Ankle swelling secondary to cardiac causes is classically worse later in the day after the patient has been walking around. The hydrostatic pressure in the small blood vessels is greater when the legs are held vertical, so increasing the accumulation of fluid in the interstitial spaces. At night, however, the legs are raised, reducing intravascular pressure and allowing flow of fluid back into the venules with reduction of the oedema by morning.

Non-cardiac causes of ankle swelling include:

- renal – due to proteinuria
- hepatic – due to low serum albumin
- protein malnutrition – due to low serum albumin
- pulmonary – due to hypercapnia and hypoxia in COPD.

Fig. 22.3 Differential diagnosis of syncope

Cause	Speed of onset	Precipitating events	Nature of recovery
Stokes–Adams attack (transient asystole; results from cerebral hypoxia occurring during prolonged asystole)	Sudden – patient feels entirely well immediately before syncope	Often none	Rapid, often with no sequelae
Tachycardia – VT or very rapid SVT	Sudden	Often none	Rapid
AS and HCM	Sudden	Exertion, sometimes no warning	Rapid
Vasovagal syncope	Preceded by dizziness,	Sudden pain, emotion, micturition Patient often feels nauseated or vomits	Rapid
Orthostatic hypotension	Rapid onset after standing	Standing up suddenly, prolonged standing, use of antihypertensive or antianginal agents	May feel nauseated
Carotid sinus hypersensitivity	Dizziness or no warning	Movement of the head	May feel nauseated
Neurological (may be associated with convulsions during the period of unconsciousness) – epileptiform seizure or cerebrovascular event	May have classical aura or focal neurological signs, rapid onset	Often none (certain types of flashing lights or alcohol withdrawal may precipitate epilepsy)	Often drowsy, may have residual neurological deficit
Pulmonary embolus	Chest pain, dyspnoea, or no warning	None (but ask about recent travel, hospitalization, etc.)	May have dyspnoea or pleuritic chest pain
Hypoglycaemia (may be associated with convulsions during the period of unconsciousness)	Slower onset, nausea, sweating, tremor	Exercise, insulin therapy, missing meals	Often drowsy

AS, aortic stenosis; HCM, hypertrophic cardiomyopathy; SVT, supraventricular tachycardia; VT, ventricular tachycardia.

SYSTEMS REVIEW

It is very important to learn the skill of taking a rapid, but detailed, systems review. This part of the history consists of direct questions covering the important symptoms of disease affecting systems other than the one covered in the presenting complaint. Learn the questions by heart so that you automatically ask them every time you take a history (note that this is only time-consuming if the doctor has trouble remembering the questions to ask).

Respiratory system

Cough

Cough may suggest the presence of infection; a common cause of arrhythmias. Cough is also a symptom of cardiac failure.

Haemoptysis

Haemoptysis is a feature of pulmonary embolism, pulmonary oedema (sputum may be pink and frothy), pulmonary hypertension secondary to mitral valve disease and pulmonary infection.

Fig. 22.4 Causes of palpitations

Rhythm	Precipitating factors	Relieving factors
Sinus tachycardia	Anxiety, exertion, thyrotoxicosis, anaemia	Rest or specific treatment of underlying condition
Atrial fibrillation	Ischaemia, thyrotoxicosis, hypertensive heart disease, mitral valve disease, alcoholic heart disease, pulmonary sepsis or embolism, idiopathic	Antiarrhythmic agents or treatment of the underlying disorder
Atrial flutter	Thyrotoxicosis, sepsis, alcohol, caffeine, pulmonary embolus, idiopathic	Antiarrhythmic agents or treatment of the underlying cause
AV and AV nodal re-entry tachycardias	Caffeine, emotion, alcohol, or no obvious cause	Vasovagal stimulation, ablation of re-entry pathway or antiarrhythmic drugs
VT	Ischaemia, ventricular dysplasia	Antiarrhythmic agents, treatment of the underlying cause or ablation of focus of arrhythmia
Bradyarrhythmias (AV nodal block or sinus node disease)	Often none (overtreatment of tachycardia with antiarrhythmic agents)	Stop antiarrhythmic agent or insert permanent pacemaker

AV, atrioventricular; VT, ventricular tachycardia.

Wheeze

This is classically seen in asthmatics (remember that asthmatics cannot take β-blockers), but is also a feature of cardiac asthma as a sign of pulmonary oedema. Patients who have chronic obstructive airways disease may complain of wheeze; these patients have often been heavy smokers and are, therefore, at risk of cardiac disease.

Gastrointestinal system

Appetite

Appetite is often reduced in cardiac failure because patients are too breathless to eat; this and other factors lead to cardiac cachexia.

Weight loss or gain

Oedema can cause marked weight gain. Severe cardiac failure or infective endocarditis can cause weight loss.

Nausea and vomiting

Nausea and vomiting often complicates an acute myocardial infarction (MI), vasovagal syncope and drug toxicity (e.g. digoxin toxicity).

Indigestion

This may be confused for ischaemic cardiac pain and vice versa.

Diarrhoea and constipation

Diarrhoea may lead to electrolyte imbalance affecting cardiac rhythm or may be a sign of viral illness leading to myocarditis or pericarditis.

Central nervous system

Headache

Headache may be a side effect of cardiac drugs (e.g. nitrates and calcium channel blockers).

- Smoking – a recognized risk factor in cardiovascular disease
- Use of illegal drugs – intravenous drug abuse is associated with a high risk of infective endocarditis. The organisms involved are unusual (e.g. *Staphylococcus aureus*, *Candida albicans*, Gram-negative organisms and anaerobes). Cocaine abuse is associated with coronary artery spasm and increased myocardial oxygen demand resulting, in some cases, in myocardial ischaemia and infarction. Long-term use of cocaine may result in dilated cardiomyopathy
- Alcohol intake – heavy alcohol consumption has many cardiac effects (Fig. 22.6). Alcohol is a potent myocardial depressant when taken in excess over a long period.
- It should also aim to establish the patient's support network – who is at home, does the patient need any help with the activities of daily living from friends or family, or are they in need of outside help from social services?
- Exercise capacity – it is useful to gauge how much the patient can do and what limits their activity.

Objectives

By the end of this chapter you should:

- be able to examine the cardiovascular system to elicit signs of cardiovascular disease
- be able to differentiate systolic and diastolic murmurs and understand the valve lesions associated with them
- understand the clinical manifestations of cardiac disease outside the cardiovascular system.

This chapter provides information on how to examine the cardiovascular system. The method of examination remains the same whether you are sitting for finals or for the membership examination, so you should learn it properly once and for all. Remember that cardiovascular cases are among the most popular used in short-case examinations.

HOW TO BEGIN THE EXAMINATION

Ensure that the patient is comfortable at all times and establish rapport to put them at ease. You need to expose the patient in order to examine them properly but cover the patient to maintain modesty, and as soon as you have finished the examination.

Always start by introducing yourself and shaking hands gently (many elderly patients have painful arthritic joints – never make patients wince when you shake hands with them). Ask if you can examine the patient's chest and heart.

Position the patient correctly. The patient should remove all clothing from the waist upward – it is acceptable for a female patient to cover her breasts when you are not observing or examining the praecordium.

The patient should be sitting comfortably against the pillows with his or her back at 45° with the head supported so that the neck muscles are relaxed – the only two circumstances when you may deviate from this position are:

- if the patient has such bad pulmonary oedema that he or she needs to sit bolt upright
- if the jugular venous pressure (JVP) is not raised, a more recumbent position will fill the jugular vein and allow examination of the venous pressure waveform.

OBSERVATION

As soon as you see the patient, and during your introductions, you should be observing the patient and his or her surroundings. Once the patient has been positioned, expose the chest, step to the end of the bed and observe for a few seconds.

Observation is an art and you will be surprised by how much information you can obtain and remember after only a few seconds. In many cases this part of the examination provides valuable clues about the diagnosis. The secret to this is knowing what to look for.

Look at the patient's face for the following signs:

- Breathlessness, central cyanosis
- Malar flush of mitral stenosis
- Corneal arcus or xanthelasma – suggestive of hypercholesterolaemia
- Any signs of congenital abnormality, such as the classic appearance of Down's syndrome or Turner's syndrome.

197

Additional information can be obtained by looking at the conjunctivae. The presence of conjunctival haemorrhages suggests infective endocarditis; the presence of conjunctival pallor suggests anaemia.

Look briefly in the mouth for:

- tar staining of the teeth – seen in heavy smokers
- central cyanosis.

EXAMINATION OF THE JUGULAR VENOUS PRESSURE

This is sometimes difficult, so make things easier by ensuring the patient is in the correct position (at 45 ° with the head supported and the neck muscles relaxed).

The internal jugular vein is used because it has no valves and is not subject to as much muscular compression as the external jugular vein. The JVP gives an indication of the right atrial pressure (Fig. 23.4). The normal JVP is less than 3 cmH$_2$O (measured as the vertical distance above the angle of Louis). This rests at the level of the clavicle so the normal JVP waveform is not usually visible or, if it is seen, the pulsation is just above the clavicle. It can be visualized by lying the patient flat. In sinus rhythm, there are two waves:

1. 'a' just preceding the carotid pulse – this is absent in atrial asystole and AF
2. 'v', which is accentuated in tricuspid regurgitation.

Occasional 'cannon' waves are seen in heart block when the right atrium contracts against a closed tricuspid valve.

The differences between the JVP and carotid pulse are highlighted in Fig. 23.5.

Kussmaul's sign

Normally, the JVP falls with inspiration because the pressure in the thoracic cavity is negative. In constrictive pericarditis or cardiac tamponade the JVP increases with inspiration; this is known as Kussmaul's sign.

EXAMINATION OF THE PRAECORDIUM

Palpation

The following sequence of palpation should be observed:

- Palpate the apex beat, defined as the lowest and most lateral point at which the cardiac impulse can be felt. Always start palpating in the axilla and move anteriorly until you feel the apex beat. If you start palpating anteriorly it is possible to miss a grossly displaced apex. Define the character of the apex beat (Fig. 23.6).
- Palpate the left lower sternal edge to feel for a right ventricular heave (a sign of pulmonary

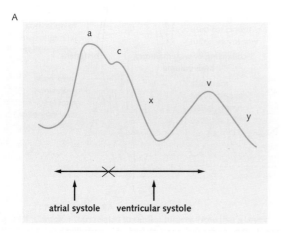

A

atrial systole   ventricular systole

Fig. 23.4B Causes of the waves and descents in the JVP

Wave or descent	Cause
a wave	Right atrial systole, which results in venous distension
c wave	Increasing right ventricular pressure just before the tricuspid valve closes producing an interruption in the x descent
x descent	Atrial relaxation and pulling down of the base of the atrium caused by right ventricular contraction
v wave	Right atrial filling during right ventricular systole
y descent	Fall in right atrial pressure as the tricuspid valve opens

Fig. 23.4 (A) Jugular venous pressure (JVP) waveform. (B) Causes of the waves and descents in the JVP.

Fig. 23.5 Differences between the jugular venous pressure (JVP) and carotid pulse

Feature	JVP	Carotid pulse
Character of pulse	Double pulsation: a wave occurs at end of diastole, v wave with systole	Single systolic pulse
Potential for obliteration	Can be obliterated by pressing on vein just above the clavicle	Cannot be obliterated
Effect of position	If the patient sits upright it falls	No effect
Effect of pressure on the liver or abdomen	Rises (the hepatojugular reflex)	No effect
Palpable pulsation	Usually not palpable	Palpable

hypertension or pulmonary stenosis) – use the flat of the hand pressing firmly to feel this.

- Palpate the second left intercostal space where a palpable pulmonary component of the second heart sound (P_2) may be felt (a sign of pulmonary hypertension). This is felt with the fingertips.
- Palpate the second right intercostal space where a palpable thrill of aortic stenosis may be felt – this is also felt with the fingertips.

Percussion

Percussion of the heart is rarely performed and can be excluded from the routine examination. The area of cardiac dullness is affected by lung conditions (e.g. emphysema). However, an increased area of dullness indicates cardiac enlargement or pericardial effusion. This is useful if the apex beat is not palpable.

Auscultation

When listening to the heart every murmur should be systematically excluded. You should at all times be able to explain exactly which sounds you are expecting to hear at any stage during auscultation.

Learn a systematic approach, not necessarily the one described in this chapter, but always listen to the heart in the same way.

Knowing when systole and diastole are is fundamental. Know this at all times during auscultation by keeping a finger or thumb on the carotid pulse.

The order for auscultation is as follows:

- Using the diaphragm of the stethoscope listen quickly at the mitral, tricuspid, pulmonary and aortic areas in that order – you should already know where these are; if not then learn it now (Fig. 23.7). This enables you to hear any loud murmurs and possibly begin to approach the diagnosis.

Fig. 23.6 Causes of different types of apex beat

Character	Causes
Tapping	Mitral stenosis
Thrusting	Mitral regurgitation, aortic regurgitation
Heaving	Aortic stenosis
Diffuse (the normal apex beat should be discrete and localized to an area no bigger than a 10-pence piece)	Left ventricular failure, cardiomyopathy Pericardial effusion
Double	Hypertrophic obstructive cardiomyopathy, left ventricular aneurysm

Objectives

By the end of this chapter you should:

- understand the importance of clear and accurate note keeping
- understand that all entries in the notes should be labelled with the date, time, your name and your grade
- have a framework for writing the clerking into the medical notes.

There is no single correct way to write a medical clerking, but there are several incorrect ways! Remember that doctors, nurses, physiotherapists and many other health professionals use the medical notes during the course of a patient's medical care. The notes need to last for years and your entries in them may provide valuable information to doctors looking after the patient in several years' time. It is also worth remembering that the medical notes are legal documents that might one day be used as evidence in a court of law.

The basic principles when making entries into the notes are as follows:

- Always write legibly – this sounds obvious, but notes are often illegible. Remember, if no one else can read your entry you might as well not write anything.
- A date and time should precede every entry, no matter how brief. At the end of the entry you should sign your name and, if your signature does not clearly show your name, your surname and initials should be written in capitals below it. There are no exceptions to this rule ever!
- Always be courteous to your patients and colleagues when writing in the notes. Rude or angry entries may give a certain degree of satisfaction when they are made, but serve only to make you look unprofessional when read at a later date.
- Write everything down – every time you see a patient an entry should be made in the notes, stating accurately the content and outcome of the consultation. This may sometimes seem pedantic, but most qualified doctors will be able to recall situations when careful documentation resolved a difficult situation.

DOCUMENTATION OF THE HISTORY

The history should always have the following information at the top of the first page:

- Name of patient in full plus at least one other unique identifier (e.g. date of birth or hospital number) – loose sheets often fall out of the notes so all pages of the history should have this information so they are not replaced in the notes of another patient who has the same name
- Date and time of entry
- Route of admission – if the patient is being admitted to hospital it is useful to state the route by which the admission came about (i.e. via general practitioner or accident and emergency).

Remember, the main headings of the history are:

- presenting complaint (PC or C/O – complains of)
- history of presenting complaint (HPC)
- systems review (SR)
- past medical history (PMH)
- drug history (DH)
- allergies
- family history (FH)
- social history (SH).

Fig. 24.1 Important questions to ask on systems review

System	Symptoms and signs to ask about
Cardiovascular (CVS)	Chest pain, shortness of breath, orthopnoea, paroxysmal nocturnal dyspnoea, ankle oedema, palpitations, syncope
Respiratory (RS)	Cough, sputum, haemoptysis, shortness of breath, wheeze
Gastrointestinal (GIT)	Appetite, vomiting, haematemesis, weight loss, indigestion, abdominal pain, change in bowel habit, description and frequency of stools, blood and/or mucus per rectum
Genitourinary (GUS)	Frequency, dysuria, hesitancy, urgency, poor stream, terminal dribbling, impotence, haematuria, menstrual cycle, menorrhagia, oligomenorrhoea, dyspareunia
Neurological (CNS)	Headache, photophobia, neck stiffness, visual problems, any other focal symptoms (e.g. weakness, numbness; don't forget olfactory problems), tremor, memory, loss of consciousness
Other	For example muscle pain, joint pain, rashes, depression

Presenting complaint

This should be a short list of the presenting complaint(s). There is no place in this section for any descriptions.

The purpose of the presenting complaint section is to state clearly the patient's main symptoms so that an initial differential diagnosis can be formulated. It is important that at this stage the list of differential diagnoses is large.

Examples of presenting complaints are shown in the chapter titles in the first half of this book:

- shortness of breath
- palpitations (see Ch. 4)
- collapse
- ankle swelling (see Ch. 5)
- chest pain (see Ch. 1).

History of the presenting complaint

It is here that information regarding the presenting complaint is expanded. A full description of the presenting compaint(s) in turn should be noted.

It is also important in this section to ask other relevant questions pertaining to the likely organ system(s) involved. For example:

- A patient presenting with chest pain should be asked fully about the nature of the pain and should also be asked about all relevant cardiovascular and respiratory symptoms.
- In a patient who has abdominal pain a full gastrointestinal and genitourinary systems review should be included in the HPC.

Systems review

A full systems review of the other organ systems should be entered here (Fig. 24.1).

It is not necessary to document negatives unless they are particularly relevant.

Once you have memorized the questions they will become second nature and the systems review will be very quick to do. It is worth the initial time-consuming effort to do this properly; after all, you will be taking histories for the rest of your career.

Past medical history

All previous illnesses and operations should be noted, along with details of when they were carried out and if there were any complications. Patients can be very vague about these details and you may need to speak to the relatives or the general practitioner for more information.

Drug history

All drugs taken should be documented.

Remember, you cannot say you have taken a drug history unless the doses and times of all drugs are written down accurately and legibly.

Allergies

Not only should the drugs that the patient is allergic to be documented, but the type of reaction and when it occurred should be stated.

Many patients say they are allergic to penicillin when they have only experienced some gastric discomfort while taking it. In a situation where a patient is readmitted with, for example, suspected meningitis, this might influence whether a potentially life-saving dose of benzylpenicillin can be given safely.

Family history

Any diseases that have a potential genetic causation should be documented. The family member who had the disease and whether it was the cause of death should be stated.

Social history

This should include notes on the following:

- Accurate alcohol and drug intake history
- Smoking – should be carefully documented (i.e. what is smoked, how many and for how long)
- Occupation and possible exposure to industrial dusts or chemicals
- If HIV infection is a possible differential diagnosis, a thorough history of possible risk factors. This might be embarrassing – both for you and for the patient – but it is important not to miss a diagnosis as serious as this.

DOCUMENTATION OF THE EXAMINATION FINDINGS

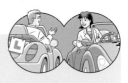

Writing a clear and logical clerking will help you to organize your thoughts in order to formulate a differential diagnosis and plan for further investigations and management. Leave yourself plenty of room as trying to fit things into a certain space may interfere with this.

There are many ways of documenting the findings on examination and it does not really matter how you do this provided a few rules are obeyed:

- The patient's name and another unique identifier are written on every sheet of paper – this should come as second nature to you.
- Any positive findings are represented in writing – diagrams can be used to aid the description, but should never be used alone to document findings because they are likely to be interpreted differently by different people (Fig. 24.2).

AT THE END OF THE CLERKING

The last section is important because it brings together all the information from the clerking. The following should be seen at the end of every clerking:

- A list of differential diagnoses with the most likely diagnosis at the top of the list.

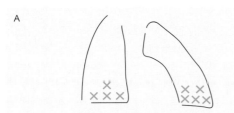
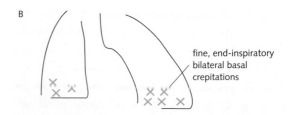

fine, end-inspiratory bilateral basal crepitations

Fig. 24.2 Potential confusion caused by lack of annotation. (A) This diagram is usually used to represent bilateral basal crepitations secondary to pulmonary oedema. However, the same diagram can be used to represent coarse inspiratory crepitations due to bronchiectasis. (B) This diagram is unequivocal and confirms the finding of pulmonary oedema.

- A list of investigations performed and to be performed – it is good practice to tick those tests that have been done already.
- A plan of action including initial drugs to be given, any intravenous fluids, physiotherapy, specific observations needed (e.g. fluid balance chart or daily weights and any consultant referrals to be made).

This reads like a long list, but you do not need to learn it. The only thing you need to remember is that if you do something that concerns a patient then write it down.

SAMPLE MEDICAL CLERKING

Hospital No: X349182
BLOGGS, Joe
11/06/35

20/06/05 19:30   63 yr old man   Referred by GP — seen in GOPD

PC   Shortness of breath

> 1. Presenting complaint should be brief, but it is necessary to include duration of symptoms.

HPC   Gradual onset of shortness of breath approximately
            6 months ago. Initially only on exertion, but
            breathlessness has deteriorated and now patient
            is breathless on minimal exertion
            (e.g. when dressing in the morning)

> 2. Mention only the relevant negatives. In this case it is important to mention the absence of haemoptysis and weight loss because of the history of cancer. It is always wise to document whether or not there is chest pain.

Associated features
            Orthopnoea
            Ankle swelling
            Cough with clear sputum and occasional flecks of blood
            Palpitations - feels heart beating rapidly and irregularly
            from time to time
            No chest pain
            No known risk factors for coronary heart disease
            NB patient unaware of his cholesterol level

Systems review
GIT: Recent loss of appetite
            No weight loss or vomiting
            No abdominal pain
            No change in bowel habit
CNS: No abnormalities on questioning
EMS: No abnormalities on questioning

PMH   Rheumatic fever when 10 years old
            Cholecystectomy 1989, no complications

DH   frusemide 40mg mane -
            started by GP last week

> 3. Always record the dose and frequency of any drugs.

Allergies   None known   Smoking - never smoked
                         Alcohol - approx 10 units/week

Fam Hx   Mother died aged 68 - stroke   SHx   Married with 2 children
            Father still alive - hypertensive   (family fit and well)
                                                                Retired accountant

O/E   Looks short of breath at rest.
Temperature 36.5°C
No central or peripheral cyanosis

> 4. Record your initial observations — they are important. 'Alert and chatty' or 'Distressed and looks unwell' tell you a lot about the patient.

CVS   Pulse 80, regular
BP 120/80 mmHg
JVP - elevated 6cm
Ankle oedema to knees
Apex not displaced
Soft low-pitched mid-diastolic murmur at apex

Hs

> 5. Always use diagrams to clarify your examination findings.

Loud P2 Marked right ventricular heave

RS: Respiratory rate 30 breaths/min
Percussion and expansion normal
Fine inspiratory bilateral basal crepitations
to mid-zones

GIT: 2cm hepatomegaly

Ascites detected
No palpable kidneys or spleen
PR not performed

CNS: No abnormalities detected on full
neurological examination

> 6. If there is no abnormality of the CNS, simply include a one-line summary.

Summary   Progressive dyspnoea in a man who has
a history of rheumatic fever and
clinical signs of mitral stenosis

Diagnosis   Pulmonary oedema and congestive heart failure
secondary to rheumatic mitral stenosis

Differential
diagnosis   Mitral stenosis of another aitiology
Paroxysmal atrial fibrillation leading to
congestive heart failure

> 7. Always include a management plan— even when you are still a student. It might not be right but you need to start training yourself to think like a doctor.

Investigations   Blood tests: FBC, V+E, LFT, TFT
Chest radiography
ECG and 24-hour ECG to rule out
paroxysmal atrial fibrilation
Echocardiography

Plan   Intravenous diuretics, initially Frusemide
80mg b.d.
Daily V&E to check effect of diuretics on
electrolytes and renal function
Daily weights and fluid input and output chart
Fluid restriction to 1500ml/24 hours
Referral to consultant cardiologist

Al-Obaidi 437

> 8. Sign your notes, including printed surname and bleep number.

Common investigations

25

Objectives

By the end of this chapter you should:

- understand how to perform an electrocardiogram (ECG)
- understand the role of non-invasive investigations in the investigation of patients with suspected cardiovascular disease
- understand the role of cardiac catheterization in the investigation of coronary artery disease, and assessment of ventricular and valvular function.

ELECTROCARDIOGRAPHY

This investigation records the electrical activity of the heart.

Lead placement

You will be expected to be able to position the electrodes correctly (Fig. 25.1) and perform an ECG by yourself, so be sure to learn this before finals.

Limb leads

There are four limb leads, one attached to each extremity:

1. Left arm (LA)
2. Left foot (LF)
3. Right arm (RA)
4. Right foot (RF).

Chest leads

There are six chest leads:

1. V1 – fourth right intercostal space
2. V2 – fourth left intercostal space
3. V3 – between V2 and V4
4. V4 – cardiac apex –you need to feel for it before placing the lead
5. V5 – anterior axillary line at same level as V4
6. V6 – mid-axillary line at same level.

12-lead electrocardiograph

The standard 12-lead ECG is derived from information given by the 10 ECG electrodes placed on the patient. It is important to know how this information is obtained when interpreting ECG findings and also when the lead positioning is incorrect.

Leads I, II and III

These are bipolar leads and were first used by Einthoven. They record the differences in potential between pairs of limb leads:

- I records the difference in potential between LA and RA.
- II records the difference in potential between LF and RA.
- III records the difference in potential between LF and LA.

These three leads form Einthoven's triangle (Fig. 25.2).

AVR, AVL and AVF

With regard to these leads:

- the letter V indicates that the lead is unipolar
- the information is obtained by connecting the electrode to a central point, which is said to have zero voltage (the reference electrode)
- AVR records the difference between RA and zero
- AVL records the difference between LA and zero
- AVF records the difference between LF and zero.

211

Fig. 25.1 Lead positions for electrocardiography. LA, left arm; LF, left foot; RA, right arm; RF, right foot.

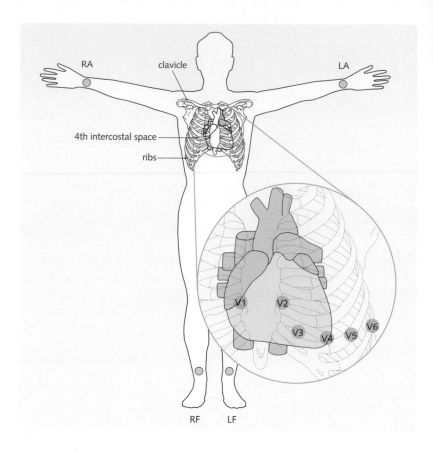

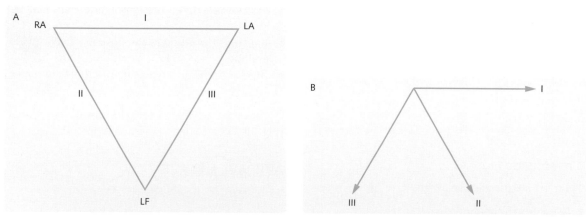

Fig. 25.2 Leads I, II and III. (A) Lead I is 0° to the horizontal, II is +60° to the horizontal and lead III is +120° to the horizontal-Einthoven's triangle. (B) Leads I, II and III are often drawn as shown here.

Chest leads

The chest leads:

- Are the precordial leads V1 to V6 and are unipolar (as seen by the prefix V).
- They each record the difference between the voltage at their location and zero.

QRS axis

The normal axis is between −30 and +90° (Fig. 25.3).

The most accurate way to calculate the axis (Fig. 25.4) is to take the lead in which the complex is isoelectric (i.e. the complex with equal magnitude

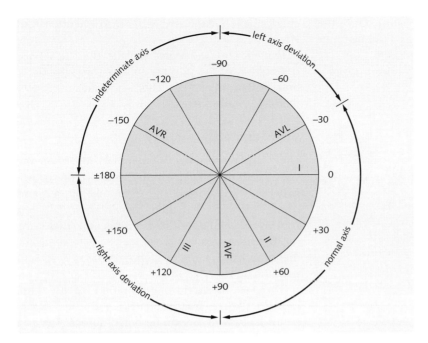

Fig. 25.3 Hexaxial reference system.

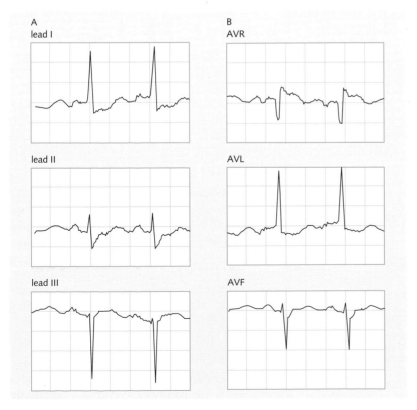

A
lead I

lead II

lead III

B
AVR

AVL

AVF

Fig. 25.4 Calculation of the axis. The QRS complex that is almost isoelectric is in lead II. Using the hexaxial reference system the two leads at right angles are −30 and +150°. The axis is −30° because the positive lead I excludes +150°.

213

in the positive and negative direction). Once this lead has been identified the QRS axis can be found because it is at right angles to this.

Causes of right and left axis deviation are given in Fig. 25.5.

A simpler way for roughly estimating the axis is as follows:

- The normal axis is in the same direction as I and II; therefore, both should be positive.
- In right axis deviation the axis swings to the right and lead I becomes negative and III more positive.
- In left axis deviation the axis swings to the left so lead III and lead II become negative and lead I remains positive.

Paper speed

The standard ECG paper speed is 25 mm/s:

- One large square (5 mm) is 0.2 s
- One small square (1 mm) is 0.04 s.

The rate is calculated by counting the number of large squares between each QRS and dividing into 300 (e.g. if there are five large squares the rate is 60 beats/min).

P wave

The P wave represents atrial depolarization, which originates in the SA node on the right atrium and spreads across the right and then the left atrium.

The amplitude of the P wave should be less than two small squares (0.2 mv) and the width should be less than three small squares (0.12 s). A tall P wave is a feature of right atrial enlargement whereas left atrial

enlargement is associated with broad and often bifid P waves.

The PR interval represents the time taken for conduction of the impulse to pass through the AV node and bundle of His. This is normally no greater than five small squares (0.2 s).

QRS complex

The QRS represents the depolarization of the ventricles, which begins at the septum. The septum is depolarized from left to right, and the left and right ventricles are then depolarized. The left ventricle has a larger muscle mass and, therefore, more current flows across it. The left ventricle, therefore, exerts more influence on the ECG pattern than the right.

The maximum normal duration of the QRS is 0.12 s (three small squares) and the QRS is abnormally wide in bundle branch block (left and right bundle branch block, Chapter 14). It is also wide when the ventricles are paced (Fig. 25.6).

ST segment

This segment is normally isoelectric (i.e. it shows no deflection from the baseline).

T wave

The T wave represents ventricular repolarization. Normally the only leads that show negative T waves are AVR and V1; the rest are positive. (A negative QRS should, however, be accompanied by a negative T wave.) Certain T wave abnormalities suggest particular non-cardiac disorders (Fig. 25.7).

QT interval

The QT interval extends from the beginning of the QRS complex to the end of the T wave and, therefore, represents time from depolarization to repolarization of the ventricles (i.e. the action potential duration).

The duration of the QT interval is dependent upon cycle length and the corrected QT interval (QTc) is normalized according to heart rate (QTc = QT/square root of the RR interval in seconds). The upper limit of normal is 0.39 s in women and 0.44 s in men.

Q waves

A Q wave is a negative deflection at the beginning of the ventricular depolarization. Small, non-significant

Fig. 25.5 Causes of right and left axis deviation	
Left axis deviation	LBBB, left anterior hemiblock, LVH, septum primum ASD
Right axis deviation	RBBB, RVH, cor pulmonale, septum secundum ASD

ASD, atrial septal defect; LBBB, left bundle branch block; LVH, left ventricular hypertrophy; RBBB, right bundle branch block; RVH, right ventricular hypertrophy.

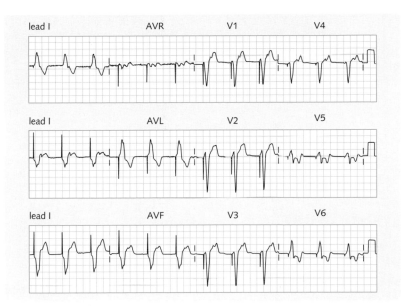

Fig. 25.6 Ventricular pacing. The sharp spikes are the artificial stimuli from the pacemaker. Each is followed by a wide QRS complex indicating the left-ventricular response. Whenever the impulse is generated in one ventricle, because of either a pacing wire or a ventricular ectopic focus, the QRS is widened. This mimics the electrical disturbances seen in bundle branch block, because the two ventricles are not depolarized in the normal sequence.

Q waves are often seen in the left-sided leads due to the depolarization of the septum from left to right. Significant Q waves:

- are more than 0.04 s (one small square) in duration and more than 2 mm in depth
- occur after transmural myocardial infarction (MI) where the myocardium on one side of the heart dies. This myocardium has no electrical activity and, therefore, the leads facing it are able to pick up the electrical activity from the opposite side of the heart. (The myocardium depolarizes from the inside out; therefore, the opposite side of the heart depolarizes away from these leads, resulting in a negative deflection or Q wave.)

U wave

This is an abnormal wave in some patients, but can appear in the chest leads of normal ECGs. It is an upright wave that appears after the T wave (Fig. 25.8); causes include:

- hypokalaemia
- hypocalcaemia.

Fig. 25.7 Electrocardiographic abnormalities in non-cardiac disease

Cause	ECG abnormalities
Hypothermia	J waves, baseline shiver artefact, bradycardia; watch out for arrhythmias as the patient is warmed up
Hyperkalaemia	Tall peaked T waves, small P wave, gradual widening of the QRS, if serum potassium very high – ventricular fibrillation
Hypokalaemia	Decreased T wave amplitude, long QT interval, U waves
Hypocalcaemia	Long QT interval, U waves
Hypercalcaemia	Short QT interval, ST segment depression
Digoxin	Downsloping ST segment (reverse tick shape), T wave inversion
Digoxin toxicity	AV block, atrial tachycardia with block, ventricular arrhythmias

AV, atrioventricular.

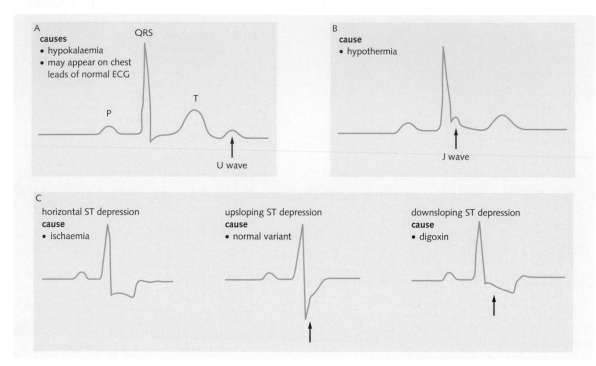

Fig. 25.8 U waves, J waves and ST segment depression.

Reporting an electrocardiograph

You will often be asked to comment on an ECG and it is difficult to remember to include everything. This exercise should be treated like the history or the examination in that you should always follow a strict routine. After a short time this will become second nature to you.

The order of examination of an ECG is as follows:

- Name of the patient and date of the ECG
- Rate (i.e. the number of large squares between the QRS complexes divided into 300)
- Rhythm (e.g. regular, irregular or irregularly irregular)
- Look at each part of the complex-P waves, PR interval, QRS complexes and QRS duration, ST segment and T waves – comment on these either out loud when you are starting to do this or in your head when you are more experienced, and comment on any abnormalities.

If there are abnormalities look to see whether they are global or territorial. Remember the territories:

- Anterior – V1–V4.
- Inferior – II, III and AVF
- Lateral – I, AVL, V4–V6.

When reporting an ECG:
- Note the patient's name and date
- Look at the rate and rhythm
- Comment on P, QRS and T waves (note shape and duration)
- Look at the distribution of changes – is it global or regional?

Exercise electrocardiography

This investigation is important in the diagnosis of ischaemic heart disease. In addition it provides prognostic information.

Indications for exercise testing

The most common indication for exercise testing is to establish the diagnosis of ischaemic heart disease

216

in a symptomatic patient. Other indications are as follows:

- After MI to evaluate prognosis and the need for further investigation or treatment
- After MI to aid rehabilitation – this gives the patient and doctor an idea of exercise capabilities.
- To detect exercise-induced arrhythmias – the increased catecholamine levels and metabolic acidosis caused by exercise potentiate arrhythmias in those patients vulnerable to this. This gives an indication of prognosis and whether treatment is required or not
- DVLA requirements, e.g. for holders of an HGV license.

Methods of exercise

The aim of the exercise test is to stress the cardiovascular system, hence it is often referred to as an exercise stress test (EST) or exercise tolerance test (ETT). All exercise protocols have a warm-up period, a period of exercise with increasing grades of intensity and a cool-down period.

The best method is treadmill exercise. Other methods, such as bicycle testing, are often less effective because many patients are not used to the cycling action and, therefore, leg fatigue often sets in before cardiovascular fatigue, resulting in early termination of the test. However, bicycle testing has the advantage that the workload can be controlled and recorded in watts.

The Bruce protocol is often used in conjunction with treadmill testing. This involves 3-min stages starting with 3 min at a speed of 1.7 miles/h and a slope of 10°. Subsequent stages are at incrementally higher speeds and steeper gradients. The final stage (stage 6) is at a rate of 5.5 miles/h and a gradient of 20°.

The modified Bruce protocol is sometimes used for patients likely to have poor exercise tolerance. An additional two stages are added to the beginning of the standard Bruce protocol. Again they are 3 min in duration and at a speed of 1.7 miles/h, but the gradient starts at 0 and increases to 5° in the first and second stage, respectively.

Patient preparation

The following should be completed before testing:

- All patients should have been seen and examined by a physician to ensure there are no contraindications to testing (see below).

- The test and its indications and risks should have been fully explained to the patient.

Certain patients are advised to stop all anti-hypertensive and antianginal medication before the test. The operator should be aware of patients still taking their medication (especially drugs affecting the heart rate such as β-blockers), because this affects the response to exercise.

Variables measured

12-lead electrocardiograph

The patient is fitted with the standard 12-lead ECG equipment. Poor electrode contact is avoided by shaving hair.

Blood pressure

Normal response to exercise involves an increase in blood pressure. An inadequate response or a fall in blood pressure with exercise indicates the likelihood of the following disorders:

- Coronary artery disease – the most common cause
- Cardiomyopathy
- Left-ventricular outflow tract obstruction
- Hypotensive medication.

Heart rate response

Heart rate normally increases with exercise. If the increase is inadequate ischaemic heart disease or sinus node disease must be suspected (also ingestion of β-blockers and calcium channel antagonists).

An excessive increase in heart rate indicates reduced cardiac reserve as in left-ventricular failure (LVF) or anaemia.

These variables are measured before, during and after exercise. Measurements are stopped once all variables have returned to their pre-exercise levels.

Test end-points

The following are appropriate indications for terminating an exercise test:

- Attainment of maximal heart rate (maximal heart rate is 220 minus age in years; in a modified Bruce protocol the submaximal heart rate is used, which is 85% of maximal heart rate).
- Completion of all stages of the test with no untoward symptoms and without attaining maximum heart rate.

Premature termination of the exercise test is indicated if any of the following occur:

- Excessive dyspnoea or fatigue
- Chest pain
- Dizziness or faintness
- Any form of arrhythmia
- Failure of blood pressure to increase or an excessive increase in blood pressure (e.g. systolic 220 mmHg)
- Failure of heart rate to increase
- ST segment depression greater than 1 mm
- ST segment elevation.

Positive exercise test

The following are indications of a positive exercise test (i.e. highly suggestive of coronary artery disease):

- ST segment depression of more than 1 mm – this should occur in more than one lead and the ST segments should preferably not be upsloping (Fig. 25.9)
- ST segment elevation
- Chest pain – provided that the pain has the characteristics of angina pain
- Ventricular arrhythmias
- Abnormal blood pressure response.

Causes of ST segment depression are listed in Fig. 25.10.

Contraindications to exercise testing

This list includes conditions in which additional stress on the heart may be very hazardous:

- Marked aortic stenosis – gradient greater than 50 mmHg with normal left-ventricular function
- Acute pyrexial or flu-like illness
- Cardiac failure
- Unstable angina
- Second- or third-degree atrioventricular block
- Patients unable to walk effectively (e.g. due to severe arthritis or peripheral vascular disease).

Despite adhering to these rules, exercise testing does have a mortality rate of approximately 0.5–1/10 000.

In all cases there should be a defibrillator at hand and all the necessary equipment for advanced cardiopulmonary resuscitation.

ECHOCARDIOGRAPHY

Echocardiography is the use of ultrasound to investigate the structure and function of the heart.

Fig. 25.9 Computer-averaged exercise ECG report showing ST depression after exercise (right-hand trace) compared with resting ECG (left-hand trace) in each of the ECG leads. There is a good tachycardia in response to exercise and the blood pressure rises to 166/84 mmHg. The ST depression is in the lateral leads V3–V6 and the inferior leads II, III and AVF. ETT, exercise tolerance test.

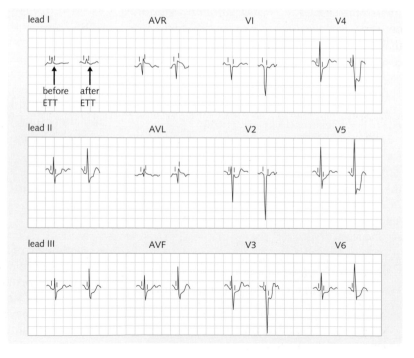

Fig. 25.10 Causes of ST segment depression

Source	Pathology
Cardiac	Ischaemia, AS, LVH, intraventricular conduction defect (e.g. LBBB)
Non-cardiac	Hypokalaemia, digoxin, hypertension

AS, aortic stenosis; LBBB, left bundle branch block; LVH, left ventricular hypertrophy.

The frequency of the ultrasound waves used is between 1 and 10 MHz (1 MHz = 1 000 000 Hz). The upper limit of audible sound is 20 kHz (1 kHz = 1000 Hz).

The ultrasound waves are generated by a piezoelectric element within the transducer. They travel through certain structures (e.g. blood) and are reflected off others (e.g. muscle and bone). The reflected waves are picked up by the transducer and, by knowing the time taken for the sound to return and the speed of the waves through the medium, the distance of the reflecting object from the transducer can be calculated.

By rapidly generating waves and detecting reflected waves a picture of the heart can be built up.

M mode echocardiography

The transducer is stationary and records only a single cut through the heart producing an image on a moving page. The result is the activity along that line seen changing with time. This mode of echocardiography is useful for:

- visualizing the movement of the mitral and aortic valve leaflets
- assessing left-ventricular dimensions and function
- assessing aortic root size
- assessing left atrial size.

Two-dimensional echocardiography

The ultrasound generator moves from side to side so a sector of the heart is visualized.

In the echocardiographic examination standard views of the heart are taken (Fig. 25.11) to provide information on:

- valve structure and function
- left-ventricular contractility

- size of the chambers
- congenital cardiac malformations
- pericardial disease.

The inadequacies of this approach are:

- the presence of lung between the heart and chest wall precludes ultrasound travel – 'poor windows'
- the posterior part of the heart is furthest from the transducer and may not be viewed adequately, particularly when searching for thrombi and vegetations.

Doppler echocardiography

This uses the principle of the Doppler effect to record blood flow within the heart and great vessels. The Doppler effect is the phenomenon where the frequency of ultrasound reflected off moving objects (e.g. blood cells) varies according to the speed and direction of movement. Colour Doppler echocardiography uses different colours, depending on the direction of blood flow, to enable the operator to assess both the speed and the direction of blood flow.

Doppler echocardiography is used for assessment of:

- valve stenosis and regurgitation
- atrial and ventricular septal defects, patent ductus arteriosus and other congenital anomalies
- pulmonary hypertension.

Transoesophageal echocardiography

Transoesophageal echocardiography (TOE) uses a flexible probe with a two-dimensional transducer incorporated into the tip. Images are obtained by introducing the transducer into the distal oesophagus.

The advantage of TOE is that images are much clearer because the transducer is in close apposition to the heart. Because of this, TOE is the investigation of choice for assessment of:

- intracardiac thrombus – transthoracic echocardiography (TTE) is unreliable
- prosthetic valve function – the planes used in TTE result in a great deal of artefact generated by the prosthesis
- valve vegetations
- congenital heart lesions (e.g. atrial and ventricular septal defects).

Fig. 25.11 Two-dimensional and M mode echocardiography. The top illustration shows a long axis view of the heart taken from the left parasternal position with the transducer placed at the left lower sternal edge. The B view shows the opening and closing of the mitral valve (MV). The normal valve gives an M shape when opening and closing with time. Left- and right-ventricular diameters are also measured with this view. The C view shows the aortic valve (AV) leaflets, which make a box shape when opening and closing with time. Left atrial and aortic root measurements can be made here. Cl, closed; IVS, interventricular septum; LV, left ventricle; O, open; RV, right ventricle.

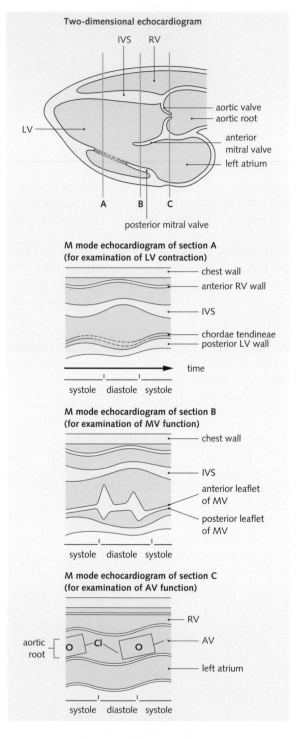

TOE imaging can be performed in multiple planes, whereas TTE is restricted to a few planes. TOE can also be used intraoperatively during cardiac surgery to provide information on valve function and left-ventricular function.

Stress echocardiography

When myocardium is ischaemic it contracts less strongly and efficiently.

The patient's heart is stressed with a drug such as dobutamine, which increases the rate and force of contraction and causes peripheral vasodilatation, so mimicking exercise. With a skilled operator echocardiography images are obtained before, during and after dobutamine and areas of ischaemia are seen as areas of regional wall motion abnormality, which recover at rest.

MYOCARDIAL PERFUSION IMAGING

This investigation uses radiolabelled agents, which are taken up by the myocardium proportional to local myocardial blood flow. It is more sensitive and specific than exercise testing alone, but much more expensive. A number of radiolabelled agents are used:

- Technetium-99m-labelled agents (e.g. ^{99m}T-sestamibi). ^{99m}T-sestamibi has a half-life of 6 h and is taken up by perfused myocardium. It remains in the myocardium for several hours and imaging of the heart provides an accurate picture of regional myocardial perfusion. Because of this phenomenon, resting and exercise images are obtained on two different days with an injection of ^{99m}T-sestamibi for each day.
- Thallium-201 is also taken up by the myocardium only in perfused areas. Unlike ^{99m}T-sestamibi, thallium is continually being passed across the cell membrane (i.e. it is extruded by one cell and taken up by another). This redistribution allows for early and late images to be taken after exercise using only a single injection. The image early after exercise (or drug stimulation) shows any areas of reduced uptake and the second image a few hours later will show whether these areas have normal uptake, suggesting the presence of reversible ischaemia.

Methods of stressing the heart

There are a number of ways to stress the heart. Wherever possible, physical exercise should be used, because this is actual physiological stress.

For those patients who are unable to exercise due to poor mobility, peripheral vascular disease, or respiratory disease, pharmacological stress may be used. (Patients who have aortic stenosis or cardiac failure should not have any sort of stress testing.)

The following are commonly used agents for pharmacological stress:

- Dipyridamole – this blocks the reabsorption of adenosine into the cells, so increasing intravascular adenosine concentrations. Adenosine is a powerful vasodilator and vasodilates normal coronary arteries, but not diseased coronary arteries. It, therefore, redistributes blood flow away from diseased vessels. This relative hypoperfusion of diseased areas is picked up by radionucleotide myocardial imaging
- Adenosine – a direct infusion of adenosine may be used
- Dobutamine infusion – this drug mimics exercise by increasing myocardial rate and contractility.

Note that both dipyridimole and adenosine are contraindicated in patients who have bronchospasm.

Either myocardial perfusion imaging or stress echocardiography are used in the following situations:
- If the exercise ECG is equivocal and confirmation of reversible ischaemia is required before coronary angiography.
- If the patient cannot perform an exercise ECG due to poor mobility – in this situation a perfusion scan is performed using drugs to stress the heart.
- In all other situations an exercise ECG is the first investigation.

Multigated acquisition scanning

Multigated acquisition (MUGA) scanning is a radionucleotide technique for evaluating cardiac function.

Technetium-99 m label is used to label the patient's red blood cells.

The amount of radioactivity detected within the left ventricle is proportional to its volume and its degree of contraction during systole will affect this.

The imaging of the cardiac blood pool is synchronized to the ECG trace and each image is identified by its position within the cardiac cycle.

Hundreds of cycles are recorded and an overall assessment of the left-ventricular ejection fraction can be made using the averaged values for end-systolic and end-diastolic volume.

MAGNETIC RESONANCE IMAGING

Magnetic resonance imaging (MRI) will soon be widely used in cardiology. It has a number of advantages:

- It is non-invasive.
- It can be gated by an ECG trace, so producing still images from each stage of the cardiac cycle.
- It does not expose the patient to ionizing radiation.

Depending on which imaging mode is used, MRI has a number of uses:

- In ischaemic heart disease, myocardial perfusion and scar (infarcted) tissue can be assessed using contrast techniques. The coronary arteries can be directly visualized, although, at present, the resolution of this is limited by cardiac and respiratory motion. Also myocardial function before and after pharmacological stress can be assessed.
- It is the gold standard for assessment of cardiomyopathy.
- In structural heart disease MRI can provide a very good spatial resolution and, therefore, detailed structural information.

POSITRON EMISSION TOMOGRAPHY

Positron emission tomography provides images of the metabolic processes of the myocardium. It is used to assess myocardial viability in patients when conventional techniques (radionucleotide perfusion scanning and coronary angiography) have given equivocal results.

CARDIAC CATHETERIZATION

This invasive investigation is used when non-invasive techniques are unable to give adequately detailed information on a cardiac lesion.

Technique

Access to the right side of the heart (right heart catheter) is gained by one of the great veins (e.g. femoral vein).

Access to the left side of the heart is gained by a peripheral artery (e.g. femoral or radial artery).

In either case the vessel is punctured using a Seldinger needle (a large hollow needle) and a guide-wire is passed through the centre of the needle and into the heart using X-ray guidance. Hollow catheters can then be passed over the wire into the great vessels or the desired chamber where a number of investigations may be carried out:

- The pressure in the chamber or vessel can be recorded.
- Oxygen saturation of the blood at that location can be measured.
- Radio-opaque dye can be injected via the catheter to provide information, depending on the location of the catheter – if in the ostia of the coronary arteries the anatomy and patency of the coronary arteries can be assessed (coronary angiography); if in the left ventricle the contractility of the ventricle can be assessed by visualizing the manner in which the dye is expelled from the ventricular cavity; if in the aortic root the size and tortuosity of the aortic root can be seen by the outline of the dye within it.

Left heart catheterization and coronary angiography

Indications

This is indicated for patients who:

- have a positive exercise test or myocardial perfusion scan
- give a good history of and have multiple risk factors for ischaemic heart disease
- have had a cardiac arrest
- have had a cardiac transplantation – there is a high incidence of atherosclerosis after transplant and yearly angiograms are performed
- occupational reasons – for patients who have chest pain even if non-invasive tests are negative (e.g. airline pilots).

Note that the list of indications is much more complicated than this, but you only need to have a general idea of the common indications.

Patient preparation

The following must be completed before the procedure:

- a detailed history to ensure that the indications are appropriate and that the patient has no other serious diseases that may affect the decision to proceed. Any history of allergy to iodine must be noted
- examination of the patient to ensure that he or she is well. Peripheral pulses must all be felt for and their absence or presence noted. If the femoral approach is to be used the groin area will need to be shaved just before the procedure
- the procedure must be carefully explained to the patient
- the risks must be explained
- informed consent is obtained.

Left ventriculography

This is performed to assess left-ventricular function. Dye is injected rapidly to fill the left ventricle and X-ray images are obtained of ventricular contraction.

Coronary angiography

The left and right coronary ostia are located in turn and dye is gently injected into the arteries. Several images are obtained of each artery from different angles so a detailed picture of the anatomy of the arteries can be obtained. Images are recorded using X-ray video recording or cine camera.

Complications of coronary angiography

The average mortality and serious complication rate of coronary angiography is 1/1000 cases. The following complications may occur:

- Haemorrhage from the arterial puncture site – this is more common at the femoral site than if the procedure is performed via the radial artery. Firm pressure should be applied to the site of bleeding and a clotting screen performed; rarely operative repair is necessary.
- Formation of a pseudoaneurysm – this results from weakening of the femoral artery wall and may require surgical repair.
- Infection of the puncture site or rarely septicaemia may occur. Blood cultures and intravenous antibiotics may be required.
- Dye reaction – which may range from mild urticaria and a pyrexia to full-blown anaphylactic shock.
- Thrombosis of the artery used – this results in a cold blue foot or hand and necessitates peripheral angiography and a referral to the vascular surgeons.
- Arrhythmias – these may occur during the angiography due to coronary arterial spasm or occlusion by the catheter. Any form of arrhythmia may occur (ventricular arrhythmias are more common).
- Pericardial tamponade – this is rare and occurs as a result of coronary artery tear or left-ventricular tear. The patient becomes acutely cyanosed and hypotensive. Pericardial aspiration is required urgently.
- Displacement of atherosclerotic fragments, which then embolize more distally, resulting in MI, cerebrovascular emboli, ischaemic toes, etc.

Cardiac catheterization and coronary angiography are mandatory before a patient can undergo a coronary artery bypass operation. They provide detailed information on the severity and location of coronary atherosclerotic lesions, without which surgery cannot be undertaken. Older patients undergoing valve replacement surgery also have coronary angiography before surgery to exclude coexistent coronary artery disease. If this is found, coronary artery bypass may be undertaken at the same time as valve replacement.

CT CORONARY ANGIOGRAPHY

The advent of rapid acquisition of images has led to the use of computed tomography (CT) as a non-invasive alternative for imaging the coronary arteries. It is likely that this will be used more extensively in patients with a low or medium probability of coronary artery disease. However, for patients likely to need coronary artery intervention, cardiac catheterization will remain the investigation of choice.

It is helpful to have a working knowledge of the common cardiac investigations so that you can explain to patients what is involved and how the findings may guide further treatment.

SELF-ASSESSMENT

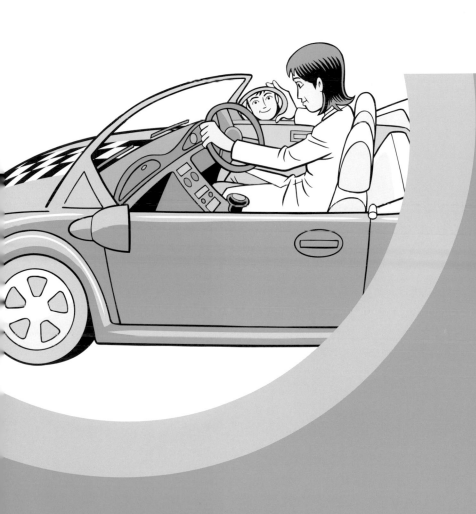

Multiple-choice questions (MCQs)

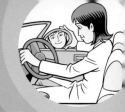

Indicate whether each answer is true or false.

1. The following are signs of right-ventricular failure:
   a. Hypotension.
   b. Hepatomegaly.
   c. Raised jugular venous pressure.
   d. Bilateral basal crepitations.
   e. Mid-diastolic murmur.

2. The following chest radiograph signs suggest left-ventricular failure:
   a. Cardiomegaly.
   b. Upper lobe blood diversion.
   c. Pleural effusion.
   d. Oligaemic lung fields.
   e. Kerley B lines.

3. The following are contraindications for the use of β-blockers (β-adrenoceptor antagonists):
   a. Cardiac failure.
   b. Asthma.
   c. Peripheral vascular disease.
   d. Diabetes mellitus.
   e. Hypotension, blood pressure less than 90/60 mmHg.

4. The differential diagnosis for chest pain includes:
   a. Myocardial infarction.
   b. Oesophagitis.
   c. Pulmonary embolus.
   d. Cholecystitis.
   e. Aortic dissection.

5. Dissection of the thoracic aorta may give the following:
   a. Hypotension.
   b. ST elevation on the ECG.
   c. Raised jugular venous pressure.
   d. Hemiplegia.
   e. A loud murmur radiating from the apex to the axilla.

6. The following are causes of acute life-threatening dyspnoea:
   a. Myocardial infarction.
   b. Pulmonary embolus.
   c. Pneumothorax.
   d. Ventricular or supraventricular tachyarrhythmia.
   e. Bacterial endocarditis.

7. The following are clinical signs found in infective endocarditis:
   a. Clubbing.
   b. Haematuria.
   c. Pyrexia.
   d. Rashes.
   e. Focal neurological defect.

8. The following are risk factors for ischaemic heart disease:
   a. Hypertension.
   b. Moderate alcohol intake.
   c. Female sex.
   d. Hypercholesterolaemia.
   e. Increasing age.

9. The following may exacerbate angina:
   a. Sleep.
   b. Tachyarrhythmia.
   c. Anaemia.
   d. High altitude.
   e. Cold air.

10. The following are classical features of cardiac syncope:
    a. Gradual onset.
    b. Warning symptoms.
    c. Rapid recovery.
    d. Residual neurological deficit.
    e. Precipitated by sudden turning of the head.

11. The following are causes of a pansystolic murmur:
    a. Mitral regurgitation.
    b. Aortic regurgitation.
    c. Tricuspid regurgitation.
    d. Atrial septal defect.
    e. Aortic stenosis.

12. The following are true of mitral regurgitation.
    a. A mid-diastolic sound may be heard.
    b. It may occur suddenly post myocardial infarction.
    c. The apex is often displaced.
    d. Atrial fibrillation may be a complicating factor.
    e. Chest radiography is the best diagnostic test.

13. **The following conditions require antibiotic prophylaxis before dental procedures:**
    a. Prosthetic aortic valve.
    b. Ventricular septal defect.
    c. Mitral valve prolapse with coexistent mitral regurgitation.
    d. Enlarged left ventricle.
    e. A history of infective endocarditis in the past.

14. **The following are complications of hypertension:**
    a. Renal failure.
    b. Cardiac failure.
    c. Diabetes mellitus.
    d. Cerebrovascular event.
    e. Ischaemic heart disease.

15. **The following should be considered as possible signs of a positive exercise test:**
    a. ST segment depression.
    b. Exercise-induced hypotension.
    c. Exercise-induced ventricular tachycardia.
    d. Lack of adequate tachycardic response to exercise.
    e. Leg pain at peak exercise.

16. **The following are recognized causes of atrial fibrillation:**
    a. Ischaemic heart disease.
    b. Hyperthyroidism.
    c. Pulmonary embolus.
    d. Jaundice.
    e. Septicaemia.

17. **The following are indications for anticoagulating a patient who has atrial fibrillation with warfarin:**
    a. Age under 60 years.
    b. Associated mitral stenosis.
    c. Atrial fibrillation of more than 24-h duration.
    d. A history of cerebral thromboembolism.
    e. Associated left ventricular failure.

18. **The following statements are true of adenosine:**
    a. It blocks conduction throughout the sinoatrial node.
    b. It has a half-life of approx 8–10 s.
    c. It is contraindicated in asthma.
    d. It may cause slowing of the ventricular rate in atrial flutter.
    e. It will cause slowing of the ventricular rate in ventricular tachycardia.

19. **The following are true of ventricular tachycardia:**
    a. It is a life-threatening condition.
    b. It may be caused by myocardial ischaemia.
    c. It may be caused by hypokalaemia.
    d. Amiodarone may be used to prevent recurrent episodes of ventricular tachycardia.
    e. Acute ongoing ventricular tachycardia should be treated initially with drugs.

20. **The following are true of digoxin:**
    a. It acts to slow conduction through the atrioventricular node.
    b. It is contraindicated in Wolff–Parkinson–White syndrome.
    c. It may cardiovert a re-entry supraventricular tachycardia to sinus rhythm.
    d. Its main route of excretion is the liver.
    e. It has a very short half-life.

21. **The following are signs of coarctation of the aorta:**
    a. Radiofemoral delay in the pulses.
    b. Rib notching.
    c. Bruits heard over the scapula.
    d. Ankle oedema.
    e. Atrial fibrillation.

22. **The following statements about infective endocarditis are true:**
    a. The most common causative organisms in Western countries are the *Streptococcus viridans* group.
    b. Fungal infections are commonly seen on the aortic valve.
    c. *Staphylococcus aureus* is associated with a benign slowly progressive disease.
    d. Enterococci are very rare.
    e. Gram-negative bacteria and diphtheroids are encountered soon after valve operations.

23. **Functions of the recovery position include:**
    a. To prevent the tongue from obstructing the airway.
    b. To prevent neck injury.
    c. To minimize the risk of aspiration of gastric contents.
    d. To maintain a straight airway.
    e. To enable cardiopulmonary resuscitation to be carried out.

24. **Complications of prosthetic heart valves are as follows:**
    a. Thromboembolic events.
    b. Dehiscence of the valve ring.
    c. Increased risk of infective endocarditis.
    d. Failure of the valve 5 years after placement.
    e. Need for anticoagulation in patients who have porcine valves.

25. **The following statements are true of thiazide diuretics:**
    a. They act at the level of the distal convoluted tubule.
    b. They may cause gout.
    c. Diabetic control may deteriorate.
    d. Hypokalaemia may occur.
    e. They cause ototoxicity.

26. **The following drugs have been shown to reduce the mortality rate for patients who have cardiac failure:**
    a. Diuretics.
    b. Angiotensin-converting enzyme inhibitors.
    c. Spironolactone.
    d. Metolazone.
    e. β-Blockers (β-adrenoceptor antagonists).

27. **The following are examples of cyanotic congenital cardiac disease:**
    a. Ventricular septal defect.
    b. Patent ductus arteriosus.
    c. Tetralogy of Fallot.
    d. Congenital aortic stenosis.
    e. Transposition of the great arteries.

28. **Cardiac causes of clubbing are as follows:**
    a. Uncomplicated atrial septal defect.
    b. Chronic infective endocarditis.
    c. Atrial fibrillation.
    d. Acute endocarditis.
    e. Empyema.

29. **Characteristic features of the jugular venous pulse are as follows:**
    a. It has a single pulsation.
    b. The v wave coincides with ventricular systole.
    c. It falls if the patient becomes more upright.
    d. It cannot be obliterated.
    e. There is no a wave in atrial fibrillation.

30. **After a myocardial infarction a patient should, if possible, be discharged on the following drugs:**
    a. A statin.
    b. Aspirin.
    c. A calcium channel blocker.
    d. An angiotensin-converting enzyme inhibitor.
    e. A β-blocker (β-adrenoceptor antagonist).

31. **The following are possible causes of electromechanical dissociation:**
    a. Pulmonary embolus.
    b. Tension pneumothorax.
    c. Hypertension.
    d. Dehydration.
    e. Hypokalaemia.

32. **The following are true of hypertrophic obstructive cardiomyopathy:**
    a. The heart is always enlarged.
    b. Patients may present with dyspnoea and/or syncope.
    c. There may be a systolic murmur on auscultation.
    d. The disease is genetically acquired.
    e. Echocardiography is often diagnostic.

33. **Mitral stenosis has the following signs:**
    a. A displaced apex beat.
    b. Malar flush.
    c. A pansystolic murmur best heard at the apex.
    d. An early diastolic murmur best heard with the diaphragm of the stethoscope.
    e. A mid-diastolic murmur best heard with the bell of the stethoscope.

34. **The following are recognized side effects of amiodarone:**
    a. Hyperthyroidism.
    b. Hepatic dysfunction.

c. Xanthopsia.
d. Peripheral neuropathy.
e. Pulmonary fibrosis.

35. **The following are characteristic of pericarditis:**
    a. The chest pain is dull in nature.
    b. There may be an associated pericardial effusion.
    c. The pericardial rub may come and go.
    d. The ECG usually shows regional ST elevation.
    e. The ST elevation is concave.

36. **The following are features of significant aortic stenosis:**
    a. Sudden death.
    b. An exercise test is contraindicated.
    c. The murmur is best heard at the left second intercostal space.
    d. The patient may present with angina.
    e. The murmur is ejection systolic.

37. **A median sternotomy scar may be used for the following operations:**
    a. Coronary artery bypass grafting.
    b. Aortic valve replacement.
    c. Closed mitral valvotomy.
    d. Mitral valvuloplasty.
    e. Heart transplantation.

38. **The following drugs are used in the treatment of hypertension:**
    a. Atenolol.
    b. Doxazosin.
    c. Enalapril.
    d. Bendroflumethiazide (bendrofluazide).
    e. Nicorandil.

39. **Features of an atrial septal defect include:**
    a. Fixed splitting of the second heart sound.
    b. A harsh machinery murmur heard at the left lower sternal edge.
    c. Increased pulmonary blood flow.
    d. Possible development of Eisenmenger's syndrome.
    e. Central cyanosis from an early age.

40. **Complications of myocardial infarction include:**
    a. Cardiac failure.
    b. Mitral regurgitation.
    c. Cerebrovascular event.
    d. Myocardial rupture.
    e. Gastrointestinal bleed.

41. **The following drugs have been shown to reduce the mortality rate after myocardial infarction:**
    a. Streptokinase.
    b. Nitrates.
    c. Heparin.
    d. Aspirin.
    e. Angiotensin-converting enzyme inhibitors.

42. **Features of pulmonary embolism include:**
    a. Chest pain.
    b. Haemoptysis.

c. Hypoxia.
d. Hypertension.
e. Left bundle branch block.

43. **Features of thoracic aortic dissection on chest radiograph may include:**

    a. Cardiomegaly.
    b. Pleural effusion.
    c. Widened mediastinum.
    d. Pulmonary oligemia.
    e. Kerley B lines.

44. **ST elevation may be associated with:**

    a. Pericarditis.
    b. Unstable angina.
    c. Thoracic aortic dissection.
    d. Pulmonary embolism.
    e. Mediastinitis.

45. **Hypoxia with hypercapnoea is detected on arterial blood gas analysis in:**

    a. Acute myocardial infarction.
    b. Acute pulmonary oedema.
    c. Pneumothorax.
    d. Mild asthma.
    e. Chronic obstructive airway disease.

46. **Clinical features suggesting pneumothorax include:**

    a. Sudden-onset chest pain.
    b. Tracheal deviation to the affected side.
    c. Hypotension.
    d. Atrial fibrillation.
    e. Hyper-resonant percussion note.

47. **Causes of metabolic acidosis include:**

    a. Large pneumothorax.
    b. Acute left-ventricular failure.
    c. Chronic obstructive airway disease.
    d. Carbon monoxide (CO) poisoning.
    e. Pneumonia.

48. **Clinical features suggesting syncope of cardiac origin include:**

    a. Ejection systolic murmur.
    b. History of exertional chest pain.
    c. History of long-distance travel.
    d. Prolonged QT interval on ECG.
    e. History of heavy alcohol intake.

49. **Rhythm disturbances leading to syncope may occur in:**

    a. Severe aortic stenosis.
    b. Septic shock.
    c. Pulmonary embolism.
    d. Acute myocardial infarction.
    e. Hypertrophic obstructive cardiomyopathy.

50. **In postural hypotension:**

    a. Blood pressure falls as a result of sinus tachycardia.
    b. There is excessive vagal stimulation.
    c. Tilt testing may be helpful.

d. May occur in long-standing diabetes mellitus.
e. May occur with antihypertensive medications.

51. **Atrial fibrillation can be differentiated from SVT by:**

    a. Palpitations are less severe and less frequent.
    b. Are precipitated by excessive coffee drinking.
    c. May be associated with chest pain.
    d. Normal resting ECG.
    e. Irregularly irregular pulse.

52. **Absent P wave on ECG characteristically occurs in:**

    a. Atrial flutter.
    b. Ventricular tachycardia.
    c. Third-degree atrioventricular block.
    d. Sick sinus syndrome.
    e. Atrial fibrillation.

53. **The following may predispose to palpitations:**

    a. Hypokalaemia.
    b. Hyperkalaemia.
    c. Hypomagnesaemia.
    d. Hypocalcaemia.
    e. Hyponatraemia.

54. **Useful investigation for peripheral oedema include:**

    a. Chest radiography.
    b. Echocardiography.
    c. Abdominal ultrasonography.
    d. Urinanalysis.
    e. Urine culture and sensitivity.

55. **Peripheral oedema due to hypoalbuminaemia may occur in:**

    a. Severe mitral regurgitation.
    b. Severe chronic obstructive airway disease.
    c. Pyelonephritis.
    d. Diabetic nephropathy.
    e. Cushing's disease.

56. **Peripheral oedema due to heart failure is associated with:**

    a. Increase in intravascular volume and extracellular water depletion.
    b. Salt retention.
    c. Severe leg oedema without a raised jugular venous pressure.
    d. Suppression of the renin-angiotensin system.
    e. May not be different from peripheral oedema due to renal failure.

57. **Early diastolic murmur may be associated with:**

    a. Aortic dissection.
    b. Acute myocardial infarction.
    c. Marfan syndrome.
    d. Pulmonary embolism.
    e. Floppy mitral valve.

58. **Mid-diastolic murmur of mitral stenosis:**

    a. Is best heard in expiration.
    b. In atrial fibrillation is associated with presystolic accentuation.

c. Is associated with a displaced thrusting cardiac impulse.
d. Can result in a slow rising radial pulse.
e. P. mitrale may be seen in the ECG.

59. Clinical features suggesting secondary hypertension include:

a. Enlarged cardiac shadow on chest radiograph.
b. AV nipping on fundoscopy.
c. Asymmetrical renal size on renal ultrasonography.
d. Buffalo hump.
e. Episodic sweating and palpitations.

60. Useful investigations for hypertension include:

a. 12-lead ECG.
b. Transthoracic echocardiography.
c. Urinary catecholamines.
d. 24-h protein excretion.
e. Abdominal X-ray.

61. ECG features of left-ventricular hypertrophy include:

a. Deep S wave in lead V6 = 25 mV.
b. R wave in V5 and S wave in V2 = 35 mV.
c. Broad QRS complexes = 12 mm.
d. T inversion in leads II, III, AVF, V5 and V6.
e. P. pulmonale.

62. Endocrine causes of secondary hypertension include:

a. Cushing's disease.
b. Addison's disease.
c. Hypothyroidism.
d. Conn's syndrome.
e. Phaeochromocytoma.

63. The following are features of endocarditis:

a. Roth spots.
b. Splenomegaly.
c. First-degree heart block.
d. Early diastolic murmur.
e. Pericardial rub.

64. Risk factors predisposing to infective endocarditis include:

a. Intravenous drug abuse.
b. Rheumatic heart valve disease.
c. Hypertension.
d. Floppy mitral valve.
e. Chronic obstructive airway disease.

65. Fever may be a feature of the following.

a. Stable angina.
b. Acute myocardial infarction.
c. Ventricular tachycardia.
d. Aortic stenosis.
e. Atrial myxomas.

66. Minor criteria for diagnosis of endocarditis include:

a. Prolonged QRS duration.
b. Raised antistreptolysin O titres.
c. Growth of *Streptococcus viridans* in sputum culture.

d. Erythema multiforme.
e. Vegetations visualized on echocardiography.

67. Clinical signs suggestive of pericarditis include:

a. Janeway spots.
b. Clubbing.
c. Pericardial rub.
d. Conjunctival haemorrhages.
e. Parasternal heave.

68. Pulsus paradoxus is:

a. An exaggeration of a normal phenomenon.
b. A blood pressure drop by >10 mmHg on expiration.
c. Characterized by alternate short and long intervals between pulses.
d. A blood pressure drop by >10 mmHg on inspiration.
e. Seen in acute severe asthma.

69. In determining the character of the arterial pulse:

a. Slow rising pulse is a feature of aortic stenosis.
b. Collapsing pulse can be a feature of mitral regurgitation.
c. Bisferiens pulse is associated with heart failure.
d. Pulsus alternans is a feature of atrial fibrillation.
e. Radiofemoral delay occurs in coarctation of the aorta.

70. With respect to Q waves on a 12-lead ECG:

a. They are always pathological.
b. They suggest transmural myocardial infarction.
c. In leads I and AVL, they suggest old inferior myocardial infarction.
d. They are due to depolarization current towards the lead.
e. They are usually transient.

71. Hyperkalaemia can be associated with the following:

a. Asystole.
b. ECG changes that correlate with potassium concentration.
c. Early changes include flattened P waves.
d. ECG monitoring is usually required.
e. Irreversible ECG changes.

72. The following features indicate a positive exercise tolerance test:

a. Development of chest pain but no ECG changes.
b. Drop in blood pressure with exercise.
c. Rise in blood pressure with exercise.
d. ST depression but no chest pain.
e. Ventricular tachycardia.

73. Recognized side effects of β-blockers are:

a. Flushing.
b. Worsening asthma.
c. Reynaud's phenomenon.
d. Impotence.
e. Renal impairment.

231

74. HMG CoA reductase inhibitors:

a. Reduce cholesterol by increasing lipoprotein lipase activity.
b. Reduce high-density lipoprotein levels.
c. Reduce cardiovascular mortality.
d. Are the drug of choice in the treatment of severe triglyceridaemia.
e. Rhabdomyolysis is a serious side effect, requiring stopping the medication.

75. The following are features of unstable angina:

a. Chest pain after 30 min walking of 1-year duration.
b. Chest pain not responding to sublingual glyceryl trinitrate.
c. Raised plasma troponin levels.
d. Has a worse outcome than non-ST segment elevation myocardial infarction.
e. Usually results from acute rupture of a coronary artery plaque.

76. Management of acute myocardial infarction includes administration of the following:

a. Aspirin.
b. Thrombolysis.
c. Statins.
d. Oxygen.
e. Angiotensin-converting enzyme inhibitors.

77. Contraindications to thrombolysis include:

a. A history of intracranial bleed.
b. Diabetes mellitus.
c. Blood pressure of 180/100 mmHg.
d. Thrombolysis within 6 months.
e. Recent gastrointestinal bleed.

78. The following are true of ventricular ectopics:

a. They can occur in otherwise healthy individuals.
b. They may occur following acute myocardial infarction.
c. They may be caused by heavy alcohol intake.
d. They usually require treatment with β-blockers.
e. They can be asymptomatic.

79. Torsades de pointes:

a. Is a form of ventricular fibrillation.
b. Is a benign rhythm disturbance.
c. Requires emergency synchronized DC cardioversion.
d. Amiodarone may be useful in preventing recurrence.
e. May be caused by hypomagnesaemia.

80. To differentiate between VT and SVT with BBB:

a. Concordance is present in VT.
b. Capture beats are seen in SVT.
c. Fusion beats are seen in SVT.
d. Intravenous verapamil can help to differentiate between the two.
e. If in doubt treat as VT.

81. The following statements regarding Advanced Life Support are true:

a. Pulseless VT requires an immediate synchronized DC shock.
b. Adrenaline (1 mg) is administered every 3–5 min.
c. Atropine (3 mg) is given as bolus every 3 min.
d. VT/VF cardiac arrest has a better prognosis than asystole.
e. ALS and not BLS is the resuscitation protocol followed in hospitals.

82. Potential reversible causes of cardiac arrest include:

a. Hypoxia.
b. Hypokalaemia.
c. Hypovolaemia.
d. Pulmonary embolism.
e. Hypothermia.

83. The following statements about AV node disorders are true:

a. Ischaemic cause is due circumflex artery disease in 40% of patients.
b. Usually reversible following anterior myocardial infarction.
c. May be associated with aortic valve endocarditis.
d. May respond to atropine.
e. Third-degree AV block is always associated with syncope.

84. Indications for permanent pacing include:

a. Trifascicular block.
b. Slow atrial fibrillation.
c. Symptomatic bradycardia due to β-blockers.
d. Left bundle branch block.
e. Mobitz type II AV block 1 week after inferior myocardial infarction.

85. The following statements of left bundle branch block (LBBB) are true:

a. QRS complexes are wider than 0.12 s.
b. Is characterized by M-shaped complexes in V1.
c. May respond to atropine.
d. New LBBB is an indication for thrombolysis.
e. May cause syncope.

86. The following are true of permanent pacemakers:

a. VVI pacing is a form of single-chamber pacing.
b. DDD pacing is useful in atrial fibrillation.
c. AAI pacing may be indicated in SA node disorders.
d. Pacemaker syndrome may occur in patients with DDD pacing.
e. The suffix R denotes rate responsiveness.

87. Management of acute left-ventricular failure includes:

a. Administration of oxygen.
b. Intravenous diuretics.
c. Oral nitrates.
d. Oral β-blocker.
e. Intravenous diamorphine.

88. Causes of dilated cardiomypathy include:

a. Long-standing untreated hypertension.
b. Amyloidosis.
c. Alcohol.
d. Hyperthyroidsm.
e. Sarcoidosis.

89. Management of hypertrophic obstructive cardiomyopathy includes:

a. β-Blockers.
b. Implantation of cardioverter/defibrillator.
c. Inducing myocardial infarction in the proximal septum (alcohol septal ablation).
d. Genetic counselling.
e. Coronary artery bypass graft surgery.

90. The following may be features of pericarditis:

a. Raised ESR and CRP.
b. Raised WBC.
c. Enlarged heart on chest radiography.
d. Echocardiography is diagnostic.
e. Atrial fibrillation.

91. Dressler's syndrome:

a. Is a type III autoimmune phenomenon.
b. May be associated with joint pain.
c. Classically occurs within 48 h of acute myocardial infarction.
d. May cause cardiac tamponade.
e. Corticosteroids are the first choice of treatment.

92. Features of constrictive pericarditis include:

a. Pulsus paradoxus.
b. Rapid x descent.
c. Preserved left-ventricular systolic function.
d. Raised jugular venous pressure.
e. Pulmonary oedema.

93. The following are clinical signs of cardiac tamponade:

a. Kussmaul's sign.
b. Pericardial rub.
c. Sinus bradycardia.
d. Low pulse volume.
e. Soft heart sounds.

94. The following are features of rheumatic valvular disease:

a. Affects mitral and aortic valves only.
b. Is caused by valve infection with group A streptococcal infection.
c. Results in cusp and commissural fusion.

d. Require antibiotics prophylaxis to prevent endocarditis.
e. Is the most common cause of mitral stenosis.

95. Features suggesting failure of treatment in endocarditis include:

a. Rising ESR and CRP.
b. Increase in temperature.
c. Embolic phenomena.
d. Microscopic haematuria.
e. A negative blood culture.

96. Indications for emergency valve replacement include:

a. Significant valve regurgitation after 6 weeks of antibiotic treatment.
b. *Staphylococcus aureus* infection.
c. Aortic root abscess.
d. Valve dehiscence.
e. Recurrent embolic phenomena.

97. Non-pharmacological management of hypertension involves:

a. Reducing salt intake.
b. Smoking cessation.
c. Regular exercise.
d. Weight loss.
e. May reduce systolic but not diastolic blood pressure.

98. The following clinical features suggest end-organ damage in hypertension:

a. Dyspnoea on exertion.
b. Dysarthria.
c. Early diastolic murmur.
d. Voltage criteria for LVH.
e. Left bundle branch block.

99. The following statements are true of tetralogy of Fallot:

a. Pulmonary hypertension is a prominent feature.
b. Squatting helps ease symptoms.
c. Includes patent ductus arteriosus.
d. Requires antibiotic prophylaxis.
e. Cyanosis persists after total surgical correction.

100. Eisenmenger's syndrome may be associated with the following:

a. Right-to-left shunt.
b. Anaemia.
c. Paradoxical emboli.
d. Clubbing.
e. Is reversible once the shunt is closed.

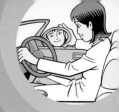

Short-answer questions (SAQs)

1. List the important steps in the management of a patient who has acute left-ventricular failure.

2. Outline the initial investigations in the accident and emergency department you would carry out on a patient who has chest pain. Give the rationale behind each test.

3. Outline the clinical features of syncope that help clarify the underlying cause.

4. Write short notes on the complications of atrial fibrillation.

5. List the peripheral stigmata of infective endocarditis.

6. What does the ECG in Fig. 1 show? Outline the treatment options.

Fig. 1

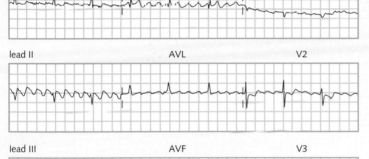

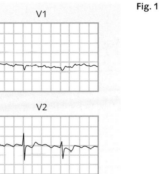

7. Outline the initial investigations in the accident and emergency department of a patient who has suspected infective endocarditis.

8. What does the ECG in Fig. 2 show? List two possible underlying causes.

Fig. 2

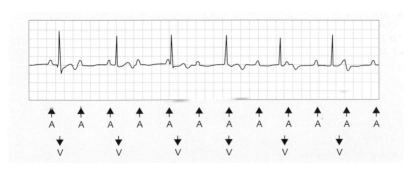

9. Write short notes on the complications of cardiac catheterization.

10. What does Fig. 3 show? Draw a flow chart to describe the acute management of such a patient.

Fig. 3

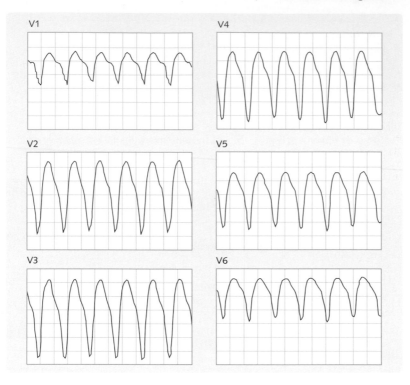

11. Describe the physical signs of mitral stenosis.

12. What diagnosis is shown by Fig. 4? Approximately how long ago did this happen?

Fig. 4

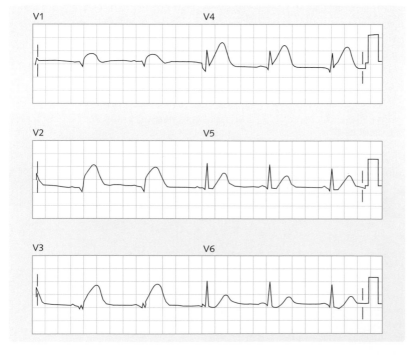

13. What are the clinical findings you would expect to see in a child who has a patent ductus arteriosus?

14. Which blood tests would you request to investigate a patient who has ankle oedema and why?

15. A 60-year-old man presents to the accident and emergency department with a 1-week history of sharp central chest pain worse on lying flat and inspiration, relieved by sitting forward. He has also noticed increasing breathlessness over the past 48h and some discomfort in both knees. Of note in his past medical history he had a myocardial infarction 6 weeks previously from which he made a good recovery. Examination reveals a low-grade pyrexia and bilateral dullness to percussion at the lung bases.

(a) What is the most likely diagnosis and why?

(b) What are your main differential diagnoses?

16. A 40-year-old publican presents to the accident and emergency department with a 4-month history of gradually increasing shortness of breath. This breathlessness is worse on exertion and on lying flat, and he now needs to use four pillows at night to prop himself up. Over the past 2 weeks he has noticed that his legs are swollen, especially at the end of each day. He denies any chest pain or palpitations. The social history reveals that he has smoked 20 cigarettes a day from the age of 16 years and that he drinks approximately 60 units of alcohol each week. He has no family history of heart disease.

(a) What diagnosis do the symptoms suggest?

(b) What is the most likely cause?

(c) Give two possible differential diagnoses?

17. Write short notes on streptokinase.

18. List the possible complications that may be seen in the first 7 days after a myocardial infarction.

19. Give four possible indications for implantation of a permanent pacemaker.

20. A young woman attends the outpatient clinic. She has a confirmed diagnosis of atrial septal defect and she is currently well. She has been told she needs antibiotic prophylaxis before certain procedures but is unsure which ones. How would you advise her?

Extended-matching questions (EMQs)

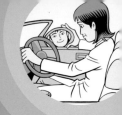

1. **Match the ECG changes below to the most likely clinical diagnosis:**

   a. ST elevation V1–V4
   b. ST depression V1–V4
   c. V2+V5 >35 mm
   d. Prolonged QT interval
   e. Concave ST elevation in all leads except AVR
   f. Short p waves and tall T waves
   g. ST elevation in leads II, III and AVF with ST depression in V2–V4
   h. Q waves in V1–V4
   i. Right axis deviation
   j. Small complexes with beat-to-beat variation.

   Instruction: For each scenario described below, choose the SINGLE most likely diagnosis from the above list of options. Each option may be used once, more than once or not at all:

   1. Family history of sudden cardiac death
   2. Pericarditis
   3. Longstanding hypertension
   4. Pericardial effusion
   5. Acute inferoposterior myocardial infarction.

2. **The drug(s) of choice for the following arrhythmias include:**

   a. Sotalol
   b. Digoxin
   c. Verapamil
   d. Flecainide
   e. Atenolol
   f. Amiodarone
   g. C or D
   h. A, C or E
   i. A and F
   j. Implantable cardioverter defibrillator (ICD) and drug treatment.

   Instruction: For each scenario described below, choose the SINGLE most likely diagnosis from the above list of options. Each option may be used once, more than once or not at all.

   1. Rhythm control for AF in a patient with known angina
   2. Rhythm control for AF in an asthmatic 35-year-old man

   3. Prophylaxis for SVT in the absence of an accessory pathway
   4. Prophylaxis for VT in a patient with poor LV function
   5. First-line rate control for AF.

3. **Choose the drug of choice for the treatment of hypertension in the scenario below:**

   a. Atenolol
   b. Perindopril
   c. Doxazosin
   d. Methyldopa
   e. Bendrofluazide
   f. Amlodipine
   g. Losartan
   h. E or F
   i. A or F.

   Instruction: For each scenario described below, choose the SINGLE most likely diagnosis from the above list of options. Each option may be used once, more than once or not at all:

   1. 70-year-old male, recent diagnosis of angina of effort
   2. 50-year-old diabetic lady who describes a dry cough having been started on ramipril
   3. 28-year-old female who is 20 weeks pregnant
   4. 37-year-old AfroCaribbean male
   5. 88-year-old female who is troubled by urgency of micturition.

4. **Which is the most appropriate next choice of cardiac investigation in the scenario described below?**

   a. Stress echocardiogram
   b. Exercise stress test
   c. Magnetic resonance imaging
   d. Computed tomography
   e. Myocardial perfusion scan
   f. Coronary angiogram
   g. Echocardiogram
   h. 24-h tape (Holter monitor)
   i. A or E
   j. No investigations are needed.

Instruction: For each scenario described below, choose the SINGLE most appropriate investigation from the above list of options. Each option may be used once, more than once or not at all:

1. 60-year-old man seen in clinic with a 3-month history of chest tightness on exertion

2. 23-year-old female who reports breathlessness on exertion and has a history of a childhood heart murmur

3. 70-year-old diabetic man who has exertional chest pain and ST depression on exercise stress testing

4. 44-year-old lady who has limited mobility and on treatment for hypertension and hypercholesterolaemia; she describes a sharp left-sided chest discomfort, but which may or may not be related to exertion. Cardiovascular examination was unremarkable

5. 40-year-old female with fast palpitations occurring for a few minutes each day. Cardiovascular examination is normal.

5. Select the most likely cause of syncope in each of the clinical scenarios listed below:

a. Hypertrophic cardiomyopathy
b. Long QT syndrome
c. Complete heart block
d. Aortic stenosis
e. Postural hypotension
f. Vasovagal syncope
g. Ventricular tachycardia
h. Vertebrobasilar insufficiency
i. Epileptic seizure.

Instruction: For each scenario described below, choose the SINGLE most likely diagnosis from the above list of options. Each option may be used once, more than once or not at all:

1. 70-year-old male with a history of three previous myocardial infarctions and coronary artery bypass grafting who describes a feeling of fluttering in the chest before losing consciousness

2. 65-year-old female with a 10-year history of diabetes and hypertension who describes dizziness on getting out of bed in the morning

3. 70-year-old male who describes a 3-week history of lethargy and shortness of breath on exertion. His heart rate is between 30 and 40 beats per minute

4. 30-year-old male with a family history of sudden cardiac death; on examination he has a jerky pulse, a double apical impulse and ejection systolic murmur

5. 35-year-old female who is previously fit and well and loses consciousness after receiving bad news.

6. From the list below select the causative factor that is most closely linked to the following complication:

a. Type III autoimmune reaction
b. Prosthetic heart valve
c. *Coxiella burnetii*
d. Recent dental work
e. Splinter haemorrhages
f. Roth's spots
g. Janeway lesions
h. Coagulase-negative staphylococci
i. Libman-Sacks endocarditis
j. C or I.

Instruction: For each scenario described below, choose the SINGLE most likely diagnosis from the above list of options. Each option may be used once, more than once or not at all:

1. Patient with rheumatic heart disease and no previous surgical history who has developed endocarditis

2. Glomerulonephritis

3. Culture-negative endocarditis

4. Failure to eradicate the infection in endocarditis

5. Retinal haemorrhage in the setting of infective endocarditis.

7. Match the diagnosis listed below with the ECG description:

a. Left bundle branch block
b. Atrial flutter
c. Accelerated idioventricular rhythm
d. Second degree heart block
e. Complete heart block with ventricular escape rhythm
f. Right bundle branch block
g. Hypothermia
h. Accessory pathway
i. Atrial fibrillation.

Instruction: For each scenario described below, choose the SINGLE most likely diagnosis from the above list of options. Each option may be used once, more than once or not at all:

1. RSR pattern in lead V1

2. P waves which have no fixed relationship with the QRS complexes. The QRS complexes are broad and the heart rate is 35 beats per minute

3. J waves

4. Delta wave

5. Left bundle branch block morphology shortly after myocardial infarction, no visible p waves, heart rate 100 beats per minute.

8. For each of the emergency situations outlined, select the definitive management plan:

a. Insertion of a temporary pacing wire

b. Primary angioplasty (or thrombolysis if not available)

c. Urgent echocardiogram with a view to pericardial aspiration

d. Urgent CT thorax with a view to cardiothoracic surgery

e. Urgent VQ scan with administration of subcutaneous low-molecular-weight heparin

f. Urgent CXR with a view to chest aspiration/drain

g. Urgent chest aspiration/drain

h. Administration of non-invasive ventilation and i.v. antibiotics

i. None of the above.

Instruction: For each scenario described below, choose the SINGLE most appropriate management plan from the above list of options. Each option may be used once, more than once or not at all:

1. 36-year-old male following a road traffic accident. Lacerated skin and apparent injury to ribs on the right side of the chest anteriorly. He is extremely dyspnoeic and there is mediastinal shift towards the left with hyperresonance of the right lung field

2. 60-year-old female with known metastatic breast cancer. Presents with a 2-week history of progressive shortness of breath, no history of chest pain. Noted to be hypotensive and tachycardic on examination

3. 75-year-old man who takes diltiazem for hypertension, presents with a 3-week history of progressive lethargy and shortness of breath. He is now dizzy even sitting still. The ECG shows complete heart block and his blood pressure is 80/50

4. 38-year-old male, recent flu-like illness. He describes left-sided chest pain, which radiates to the shoulder that has been present for 3 days constantly. The ECG shows widespread concave ST elevation but no Q waves are visible

5. 25-year-old female, 28 weeks pregnant. She has been well recently, but presents with right-sided chest pain which came on suddenly, worse on deep inspiration, and shortness of breath. She is tachycardic and hypoxic on room air.

9. From the list of drugs below, select the most appropriate choice for use in the clinical scenario described below:

a. Cardioselective β-blocker

b. ACE inhibitor

c. Angiotensin receptor antagonist

d. α-blocker

e. Calcium channel antagonist

f. Spironolactone

g. Loop diuretic

h. Hydralazine and nitrate

i. Eplerenone.

Instruction: For each scenario described below, choose the SINGLE most suitable selection from the above list of options. Each option may be used once, more than once or not at all:

1. 60-year-old male, 1 day following uncomplicated angioplasty following myocardial infarction. Already prescribed aspirin, clopidogrel, statin and β-blocker

2. 68-year-old female, presented with congestive cardiac failure, found to have LV systolic impairment on echocardiogram, much improved after 2 days of loop diuretics

3. 70-year-old male with chronic heart failure, seen in the clinic. He is in NYHA class III despite already taking bisoprolol, perindopril and frusemide at optimal doses

4. 72-year-old AfroCaribbean gentleman, whose heart failure symptoms have not improved with conventional first-line treatment

5. 40-year-old male day 1 post myocardial infarction who is taking ramipril, simvastatin, aspirin and clopidogrel. His heart rate is 80 beats per minute, blood pressure 140/70 and there are no signs of heart failure.

10. Select the most appropriate treatment option for the following conditions:

a. Thrombolysis

b. Temporary pacemaker insertion

c. Atropine

d. Central line insertion and consideration of inotropes

e. Permanent pacemaker insertion

f. Amiodarone

g. Synchronized DC shock

h. Intravenous adrenaline (epinephrine)

i. Coronary angiogram with a view to angioplasty

j. Intravenous frusemide.

Instruction: For each scenario described below, choose the SINGLE most likely management step from the above list of options. Each option may be used once, more than once or not at all:

1. Unstable angina pectoris

2. Supraventricular tachycardia with systolic blood pressure 70 mmHg

3. Ventricular tachycardia with systolic blood pressure 130 mmHg

4. Complete heart block and intermittent episodes of dizziness (no rate-slowing drugs)

5. Acute pulmonary oedema.

11. From the list of drugs below select which one you would consider discontinuing as a result of adverse effect described:

a. Aspirin
b. Isosorbide mononitrate
c. Atenolol
d. Amlodipine
e. Amiodarone
f. Bendrofluazide
g. Lisinopril
h. Clopidogrel
i. Choose not to discontinue any drug.

Instruction: For each scenario described below, choose the SINGLE most appropriate option from the above list of options. Each option may be used once, more than once or not at all:

1. Patient troubled by ankle swelling after starting treatment for hypertension

2. Acute deterioration in renal function after starting this treatment for the first time

3. Recent coronary angioplasty, itchy rash, but constitutionally well

4. Severe headache

5. Erectile dysfunction having started new treatment from GP for hypertension.

12. From the following list of congenital heart lesions, which option correlates best with the scenario described?

a. Pulmonary stenosis
b. Aortic stenosis
c. Tetralogy of Fallot
d. Coarctation of the aorta
e. Atrial septal defect
f. Patent ductus arteriosus
g. Ventricular septal defect
h. Aortic root dilatation
i. Dextrocardia
j. A or F
k. C, E, F or G
l. B, D or H.

Instruction: For each scenario described below, choose the SINGLE most likely diagnosis from the above list of options. Each option may be used once, more than once or not at all:

1. Trisomy 21
2. Maternal rubella
3. Turner syndrome
4. Marfan syndrome
5. Kartagener's syndrome.

13. Select the diagnosis that is suggested by the clinical findings described:

a. Tricuspid regurgitation
b. Pulmonary hypertension
c. Coarctation of the aorta
d. Atrial septal defect
e. Mitral valve prolapse
f. Ventricular septal defect
g. Aortic stenosis
h. Hypertrophic cardiomyopathy.

Instruction: For each scenario described below, choose the SINGLE most likely diagnosis from the above list of options. Each option may be used once, more than once or not at all:

1. Left parasternal heave
2. Double apical impulse
3. Pulsatile liver
4. Absent second heart sound
5. Mid-systolic click and late systolic murmur.

14. Match the ECG changes below to the most likely clinical diagnosis:

a. ST elevation in leads II, III and AVF with ST depression in V2–V4
b. ST elevation V1–V4
c. ST depression V1–V4
d. V2+V5 >35 mm
e. Concave ST elevation in all leads except AVR
f. Short p waves and tall T waves
g. Q waves in V1–V4
h. Right axis deviation
i. Prolonged QT interval
j. VT/VF.

Instruction: For each scenario described below, choose the SINGLE most likely diagnosis from the above list of options. Each option may be used once, more than once or not at all:

1. Hyperkalaemia
2. Pericarditis
3. Longstanding hypertension
4. Old anterior myocardial infarction
5. Acute inferior myocardial infarction.

15. Select the most appropriate treatment option for the following patients:

   a. Cardiac transplantation

   b. VVI pacemaker

   c. Coronary artery bypass surgery

   d. No treatment

   e. DDD pacemaker

   f. Propranolol

   g. Biventricular pacemaker/cardiac resynchronization therapy

   h. HMG coenzyme reductase inhibitor

   i. Angiotensin II receptor antagonist

   j. Fibrates

   k. D or F.

Instruction: For each scenario described below, choose the SINGLE most likely diagnosis from the above list of options. Each option may be used once, more than once or not at all:

1. 68-year-old diabetic male with unstable angina and three vessel coronary artery disease not amenable to percutaneous coronary intervention

2. 37-year-old female with occasional ventricular ectopics but is otherwise fit and healthy

3. 88-year-old male with intermittently fast AF requiring rate-slowing drugs now presenting with symptomatic pauses

4. 70-year-old man who is breathless on walking short distances, found to have poor LV function and broad QRS complexes. He is on optimal drug therapy and has minor coronary artery disease

5. 34-year-old diabetic female with no history of coronary artery disease, who has a fasting total cholesterol of 9.2 and normal triglycerides.

16. The most well-recognized side effect of the following drugs is:

   a. Cold extremities

   b. Leg oedema

   c. Headache

   d. Muscle pain

   e. Angioedema

   f. Dry cough

   g. Gynaecomastia

   h. Thrombocytopenia

   i. Constipation

   j. Pulmonary fibrosis.

Instruction: For each scenario described below, choose the SINGLE most likely diagnosis from the above list of options. Each option may be used once, more than once or not at all:

1. Spironolactone

2. Nitrates

3. Simvastatin

4. Carvedilol

5. Tirofiban.

17. Match a cause for pulmonary hypertension in the following patients:

   a. Mitral regurgitation

   b. Pulmonary stenosis

   c. Familial pulmonary arterial hypertension

   d. Mitral stenosis

   e. Aortic regurgitation

   f. Rheumatoid arthritis

   g. Chronic bronchitis

   h. Systemic sclerosis

   i. Pulmonary embolism

Instruction: For each scenario described below, choose the SINGLE most likely diagnosis from the above list of options. Each option may be used once, more than once or not at all:

1. 55-year-old male with a history of rheumatic fever. He has had frequent episodes of acute pulmonary oedema. On examination his pulse is irregularly irregular, he has a loud first heart sound and rumbling mid-diastolic murmur on auscultation

2. 64-year-old male who is a heavy smoker, has a chronic cough productive of grey sputum and is breathless on moderate exertion

3. 24-year-old female with no significant past medical history who presents with gradually worsening breathlessness on exertion. The only findings of note on examination are a prominent parasternal heave, loud pulmonary second sound and a third heart sound

4. 44-year-old female with a history of dysphagia, joint pain and cold extremities. On examination it was noted that she had taut skin over her fingers, and over her nose giving rise to a pursed mouth appearance

5. 38-year-old female on the combined oral contraceptive pill who describes a sudden onset left-sided chest pain which is worse on inspiration. She was recently in plaster having fractured her ankle.

18. Match a cause for heart failure in the following patients:

   a. Pulmonary hypertension

   b. Aortic regurgitation

   c. Aortic stenosis

d. Chemotherapy

e. Mitral stenosis

f. Systemic hypertension

g. Viral myocarditis

h. Alcohol

i. Atrial septal defect

j. Mitral regurgitation secondary to mitral valve prolapse.

Instruction: For each scenario described below, choose the SINGLE most likely diagnosis from the above list of options. Each option may be used once, more than once or not at all:

1. 78-year-old male with an ejection systolic murmur loudest in the aortic area, radiating to the neck and displaced apex beat

2. 56-year-old male with ankylosing spondylitis. A collapsing pulse was noted on peripheral examination

3. 65-year-old female with a mid-systolic click and a late systolic murmur

4. 19-year-old male with a recent flu-like illness. He has a third heart sound and cardiomegaly was noted on the chest radiograph

5. 44-year-old diabetic with renal impairment. Fundoscopy revealed AV nipping, silver wiring and small haemorrhages.

19. From the list below choose the most appropriate management plan for the clinical scenarios described:

a. Primary percutaneous coronary intervention (primary PCI)

b. Automated internal cardioverter defibrillator implantation

c. Heart transplantation

d. Aortic valve replacement

e. Percutaneous alcohol septal ablation

f. Percutaneous mitral valvuloplasty

g. Closure of atrial septal defect

h. Coronary angiogram

i. Coronary artery bypass graft surgery

j. Permanent pacemaker implantation

k. Mitral valve replacement

l. No intervention.

Instruction: For each scenario described below, choose the SINGLE best management plan from the above list of options. Each option may be used once, more than once or not at all:

1. A 24-year-old male is admitted to hospital with severe shortness of breath, orthopnoea and ankle swelling, an echocardiogram at admission showed an ejection fraction of 10%. He had been diagnosed with idiopathic dilated cardiomyopathy 9 months previously. Despite treatment with intravenous diuretics he remained in NYHA class IV heart failure

2. A 64-year-old male patient with angina on mild exertion undergoes cardiac catheterization. This shows a severe stenosis of the left main coronary artery, and a severe stenosis of the right coronary artery, with normal left-ventricular function.

3. 6h after successful thrombolysis for an acute inferior ST elevation myocardial infarction, a routine ECG shows complete heart block. The 48-year-old male patient is well, with a normal blood pressure.

4. A 78-year-old female with permanent atrial fibrillation presents with a history of syncope. A Holter recording confirms atrial fibrillation, and shows several pauses lasting up to 7s in duration

5. A 50-year-old male is sent for a myocardial perfusion scan to investigate a history of chest pain. The report reads '…there is a large area of reversible myocardial ischaemia in the anterior left ventricular wall…'.

20. Match a likely cause for each of the following patients who suffer from systemic hypertension:

a. Cushing's disease

b. 'Essential' hypertension

c. Doxazosin

d. Phaeochromocytoma

e. Addison's disease

f. Hyperthyroidism

g. Renal artery stenosis

h. Persistent ductus arteriosus

i. Coarctation of the aorta

j. Conn's syndrome.

Instruction: For each scenario described below, choose the SINGLE most likely diagnosis from the above list of options. Each option may be used once, more than once or not at all:

1. 74-year-old male with diabetes and known coronary artery disease complaining of headaches. On several visits to his physician his BP is recorded as 170/95

2. 23-year-old female with a complaint of progressive weight loss, palpitations, anxiety and frequent loose motions.

3. 54-year-old asymptomatic male. A left paraumbilical bruit was noted on examination

4. 17-year-old male with radiological appearance of rib notching on chest radiograph

5. 18-year-old female with progressive weight gain and development of bitemporal hemianopia.

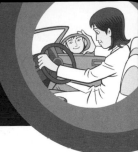

1. a. True
   b. True
   c. True
   d. False
   e. False

Comment: Bilateral basal crepitations are a feature of left-ventricular failure. Mid-diastolic murmur suggests mitral stenosis, which may lead to pulmonary hypertension and right ventricular failure, but is not a sign of it.

2. a. True
   b. True
   c. True
   d. False
   e. True

Comment: Oligaemic lung fields are a feature of pulmonary embolism.

3. a. False
   b. True
   c. True
   d. False
   e. True

Comment: Some β-blockers (e.g. carvedilol, metoprolol and bisoprolol) reduce long-term mortality in patients with heart failure. β-Blockers are not contraindicated in diabetic patients. However, these patients need to be cautioned about masking the symptoms of hypoglycaemia.

4. a. True
   b. True
   c. True
   d. True
   e. True

Comment: All can cause chest pain. You should be able to differentiate between them further by careful history taking and examination.

5. a. True
   b. True
   c. False
   d. True
   e. False

Comment: Raised JVP is not a feature of aortic dissection unless there is associated pericardial effusion/tamponade. An early diastolic murmur may result from dissection involving the annulus of the aortic valve; this is usually best heard in the tricuspid area.

6. a. True
   b. True
   c. True
   d. True
   e. True

Comment: All can cause severe dyspnoea.

7. a. True
   b. True
   c. True
   d. True
   e. True

Comment: Focal neurological defect may arise from embolization of vegetations.

8. a. True
   b. False
   c. False
   d. True
   e. True

Comment: Female risk is lower until the postmenopausal period.

9. a. False
   b. True
   c. True
   d. True
   e. True

Comment: Tachyarrhythmia increases demand whilst anemia and hypoxia reduce supply.

10. a. False
   b. False
   c. True
   d. False
   e. False

Comment: Classical cardiac syncope is of sudden onset and recovery with no warning symptoms and no residual neurological deficit.

11. a. True
   b. False
   c. True
   d. False
   e. False

Comment: Aortic regurgitation is associated with an early diastolic murmer. Atrial septal defects cause fixed wide splitting of the second heart sound and possibly ejection systolic pulmonary flow murmur. Aortic stenosis is associated with an ejection systolic murmur.

12. a. True
   b. True
   c. True
   d. True
   e. False

Comment: A chest radiograph may show enlargement of the cardiac silhouette and possibly left atrial enlargement but there are no signs that are specific to mitral regurgitation.

13. a. True
    b. True
    c. True
    d. False
    e. True

Comment: Enlarged left ventricle does not predispose to endocarditis.

14. a. True
    b. True
    c. False
    d. True
    e. True

Comment: Diabetes mellitus can result in hypertension because of renovascular complications. The reverse is not true.

15. a. True
    b. True
    c. True
    d. True
    e. False

Comment: Leg pain may indicate peripheral vascular disease.

16. a. True
    b. True
    c. True
    d. False
    e. True

Comment: Jaundice is not a cause of atrial fibrillation, although metabolic abnormalities associated with impaired liver function might predispose to AF.

17. a. False
    b. True
    c. True
    d. True
    e. True

Comment: Warfarin is not indicated in patients with AF under the age of 60 unless there is structural cardiac abnormality.

18. a. False
    b. True
    c. True
    d. True
    e. False

Comment: Adenosine slows conduction in the AV node. It has no influence on ventricular rate in ventricular tachycardia because the impulses are generated below the AV node.

19. a. True
    b. True
    c. True

d. True
e. False

Comment: Ventricular tachycardia requires immediate cardioversion to avert the possible danger of degeneration into ventricular fibrillation.

20. a. True
    b. True
    c. True
    d. False
    e. False

Comment: Unlike digitoxin, the kidneys mainly excrete digoxin. The half-life of digoxin is 36–48 h.

21 a. True
   b. True
   c. True
   d. False
   e. False

Comment: Ankle oedema and atrial fibrillation can occur with coarctation but are not clinical signs of the condition.

22. a. True
    b. False
    c. False
    d. False
    e. True

Comment: Fungal infections remain rare and are usually seen in IV drug abusers and after valve surgery. *Staphylococcus aureus* is associated with severe and destructive infection. Enterococci are the second most common cause of bacterial endocarditis.

23. a. True
    b. False
    c. True
    d. True
    e. False

Comment: The recovery position is for unconscious patients who are breathing spontaneously with good cardiac output. Head tilt should not be performed when there is a suspicion of cervical injury.

24. a. True
    b. True
    c. True
    d. False
    e. False

Comment: Bioprosthetic valves including homografts and xenografts can last an average of 10 years; mechanical valves on the other hand can last for a much longer duration. The former, however, have the advantage of not requiring anticoagulation and are more resistant to infection and endocarditis.

25. a. True
    b. True
    c. True

d. True
e. False

Comment: Thiazide diuretics do not cause ototoxicity.

26. a. False
    b. True
    c. True
    d. False
    e. True

Comment: Although essential in the treatment of both acute and chronic heart failure, diuretics (including metolazone) do not influence long-term mortality. The exception is spironolactone, which can reduce mortality by 30%.

27. a. False
    b. False
    c. True
    d. False
    e. True

Comment: Ventricular septal defect, patent ductus arteriosus and congenital aortic stenosis are examples of acyanotic congenital heart disease. The former two may become cyanotic when the pulmonary pressure rises resulting in right-to-left shunt (Eisenmenger's syndrome).

28. a. False
    b. True
    c. False
    d. False
    e. True

Comment: Empyema is a suppurative infection of the pleural cavity.

29. a. False
    b. True
    c. True
    d. False
    e. True

Comment: The jugular venous pressure has dual pulsations (a and v). Unlike carotid pulsation, the JVP can be obliterated.

30. a. True
    b. True
    c. False
    d. True
    e. True

Comment: Calcium-channel blockers are indicated only if there is suspicion of ongoing ischaemia and where β-blockers are contraindicated.

31. a. True
    b. True
    c. False
    d. True
    e. True

Comment: The cardiac output is normal in hypertension.

32. a. False
    b. True
    c. True
    d. True
    e. True

Comment: The heart is often not enlarged.

33. a. False
    b. True
    c. False
    d. False
    e. True

Comment: The left ventricle is 'protected' in mitral stenosis. A pansystolic murmur at the apex suggests mitral regurgitation. Early diastolic murmur suggests aortic regurgitation.

34. a. True
    b. True
    c. False
    d. True
    e. True

Comment: Corneal microdeposits and, rarely, impaired vision due to optic neuritis are ocular side effects of amiodarone. Xanthopsia does not occur.

35. a. False
    b. True
    c. True
    d. False
    e. True

Comment: The chest pain is usually sharp and positional. The ST changes are usually demonstrated in all leads (apart from AVR and V1).

36. a. True
    b. True
    c. False
    d. True
    e. True

Comment: The aortic stenotic murmur is best heard in the aortic area (right second intercostal space).

37. a. True
    b. True
    c. False
    d. False
    e. True

Comment: Closed mitral valvotomy is performed through a left thoracotomy incision. Mitral valvuloplasty is performed percutaneously.

38. a. True
    b. True
    c. True
    d. True
    e. False

Comment: Although nicorandil can reduce blood pressure it is used primarily as an antianginal agent and not to treat hypertension.

39. a. True
b. False
c. True
d. True
e. False

Comment: Atrial septal defect is either associated with no audible murmur or a soft mid-systolic murmur due to increased pulmonary flow. Patients with ASD are usually asymptomatic until adulthood. Cyanosis only occurs when there is shunt reversal (right to left) in untreated ASD.

40. a. True
b. True
c. True
d. True
e. False

Comment: Gastrointestinal bleeding is not a direct complication, although patients might be at higher risk of gastrointestinal bleeding because of aspirin and gastric stress ulcers.

41. a. True
b. False
c. False
d. True
e. True

Comment: Nitrates do not influence mortality but help to control chest pain due to ischaemia and reduce cardiac load. Heparin in combination with a thrombolytic agent and/or aspirin does help improve mortality; however, heparin alone does not.

42. a. True
b. True
c. True
d. False
e. False

Comment: Pulmonary embolism may be associated with hypotension, which can be severe. Right bundle branch block is a more likely association.

43. a. True
b. True
c. True
d. False
e. False

Comment: Pulmonary oligaemia is a feature of pulmonary embolism. Kerley B lines suggest pulmonary oedema due to heart failure.

44. a. True
b. False
c. True
d. False
e. False

Comment: Unstable angina is usually associated with ST depression (with the exception of Prinzmetal angina). Pulmonary embolism may be associated with sinus tachycardia, widespread T wave inversion, SI Q3 T3 pattern or right bundle branch block.

Mediastinitis may be associated with non-specific T wave changes.

45. a. False
b. False
c. False
d. False
e. True

Comment: The first four are likely to be associated with hypoxia and hypocapnoea. Severe asthma and chronic obstructive airway disease are associated with CO_2 retention.

46. a. True
b. False
c. True
d. False
e. True

Comment: Tracheal deviation occurs towards the opposite side. Atrial fibrillation may occur, but is not a feature of pneumothorax.

47. a. True
b. True
c. False
d. True
e. True

Comment: COAD is associated with respiratory acidosis due to CO_2 retention; all the others are associated with metabolic acidosis due to tissue hypoxia.

48. a. True
b. True
c. False
d. True
e. True

Comment: Long-distance travel suggests predisposition to deep-vein thrombosis and pulmonary embolism. Heavy alcohol intake can result in alcoholic cardiomyopathy and an array of cardiac arrhythmias, which may lead to syncope.

49. a. True
b. True
c. True
d. True
e. True

Comment: All these conditions may be associated with arrhythmias that may lead to syncopal attacks.

50. a. False
b. True
c. True
d. True
e. True

Comment: There is inappropriate response to vascular dilatation. Normally the heart rate increases; however, there is excessive vagal discharge resulting in relative bradycardia. Long-standing diabetes is associated with autonomic neuropathy of which postural hypotension is a feature. Vasodilators (calcium channel blockers, α-receptor blockers) can cause postural drop in blood pressure.

51. a. False
    b. False
    c. False
    d. False
    e. True

Comment: Atrial fibrillation may be similar to SVT with respect to frequency and severity of the palpitations. Excessive coffee may precipitate both and both may cause chest pain. Both may be preceded by a normal ECG (apart from SVT due to Wolf–Parkinson–White syndrome, which has characteristic resting ECG changes).

52. a. False
    b. False
    c. False
    d. False
    e. True

Comment: Although sometimes difficult to see, P waves are not absent in atrial flutter or ventricular tachycardia. P waves are independent of the QRS complexes in complete heart block and ventricular tachycardia. Intermittent P waves are seen in sick sinus syndrome. Atrial fibrillation is the only condition where P waves are not seen on ECG.

53. a. True
    b. True
    c. True
    d. True
    e. True

Comment: Electrolyte levels should always be measured in any patient who complains of palpitations.

54. a. True
    b. True
    c. True
    d. True
    e. False

Comment: Urine culture and sensitivity may help identify urinary tract infection, which is not usually associated with peripheral oedema.

55. a. False
    b. False
    c. False
    d. True
    e. False

Comment: Low albumin levels result from low protein intake, low protein production or excessive loss (gastric or renal). Pyelonephritis is not usually associated with protein loss.

56. a. False
    b. True
    c. False

d. False
e. True

Comment: Peripheral oedema is associated with salt and water retention; both intravascular and extravascular compartment volumes are increased. Raised JVP is a useful clinical method of determining central pressure in heart failure. The renin-angiotensin system is activated.

57. a. True
    b. False
    c. True
    d. False
    e. False

Comment: Acute myocardial infarction may result in rupture of the papillary muscles leading to mitral regurgitation and a pansystolic murmur. Pulmonary embolism is associated with a loud second heart sound. Floppy mitral valve is associated with a mid-systolic click and a late systolic murmur.

58. a. True
    b. False
    c. False
    d. False
    e. True

Comment: Presystolic accentuation results from atrial contraction at the end of diastole and this is absent in atrial fibrillation. Mitral stenosis is associated with a non-displaced tapping impulse. Slow rising pulse is a feature of aortic stenosis.

59. a. False
    b. False
    c. True
    d. True
    e. True

Comment: Enlarged cardiac shadow and AV nipping are features of hypertension of whatever cause.

60. a. True
    b. True
    c. True
    d. True
    e. False

Comment: Abdominal ultrasound to examine the size of the kidneys is more useful than a plain X-ray of the abdomen.

61. a. False
    b. True
    c. False
    d. False
    e. False

Comment: LVH is associated with a tall R wave in V6 (>25 mV); there might also be T wave inversion in leads I, AVL, V5 and V6. Broad QRS complexes are a feature of bundle branch block. P pulmonale suggests right atrial enlargement, which could result from pulmonary hypertension.

62. a. True
b. False
c. True
d. True
e. True

Comment: Addison's disease (primary adrenal insufficiency) is associated with low systemic blood pressure.

63. a. True
b. True
c. True
d. True
e. False

Comment: Pericardial rub suggests pericarditis.

64. a. True
b. True
c. False
d. True
e. False

Comment: IV drug abuse could predispose to infective endocarditis even in the absence of structural cardiac abnormality. Hypertension may lead to left-ventricular hypertrophy and COAD may result in pulmonary hypertension. Neither is associated with increased risk for endocarditis.

65. a. False
b. True
c. False
d. False
e. True

Comment: Stable angina and ventricular tachycardia are not associated with fever. Fever associated with aortic stenosis should raise a suspicion of endocarditis as aortic stenosis on its own does not cause fever.

66. a. False
b. True
c. False
d. False
e. False

Comment: Endocarditis may be associated with prolonged PR interval and occasionally AV dissociation. Blood culture growth of *Streptococcus viridans* is a major criterion. Similarly, vegetations seen on echo are a major criterion. Erythema nodosum and not erythema multiforme is a minor criterion.

67. a. False
b. False
c. True
d. False
e. False

Comment: Janeway spots, clubbing and conjunctival haemorrhages are features of endocarditis. Parasternal heave suggests pulmonary hypertension.

68. a. True
b. False
c. False
d. True
e. True

Comment: In pulsus paradoxus the blood pressure falls in inspiration and not expiration. The interval between pulses is normal.

69. a. True
b. False
c. False
d. False
e. True

Comment: Collapsing pulse can be a feature of aortic regurgitation, large arteriovenous malformations/fistulas or marked peripheral vasodilatation. Bisferiens pulse is associated with mixed aortic valve disease. Pulsus alternans is associated with heart failure.

70. a. False
b. True
c. False
d. False
e. False

Comment: Pathological Q waves are wider than two small squares (0.08 s) and/or >25% of the corresponding R wave. Q waves in leads I and AVL suggest a lateral infarct. The depolarization current is away from the facing lead. Pathological Q waves are permanent.

71. a. True
b. True
c. True
d. True
e. False

Comment: ECG changes are usually reversible.

72. a. True
b. True
c. False
d. True
e. True

Comment: A normal physiological response is a rise in blood pressure with exertion.

73. a. False
b. True
c. True
d. True
e. False

Comment: Flushing is often reported with calcium channel blockers. Renal impairment is not a direct side effect of β-blockers

74. a. False
b. False
c. True
d. False
e. True

Comment: Fibrates reduce cholesterol levels by inhibiting lipoprotein lipase activity. High-density lipoprotein levels may increase with statin treatment. Whereas triglyceride levels may be reduced with statin therapy, fibrates are more effective in the treatment of severe hypertriglyceridaemia.

75. a. False
b. True
c. False
d. False
e. True

Comment: Chest pain that is reproduced predictably by the same amount of effort suggests stability. Raised troponin levels suggest myocardial necrosis. Long-term morbidity and mortality is increased from unstable angina to non-ST elevation MI to ST elevation MI.

76. a. True
b. True
c. False
d. True
e. False

Comment: Statins and ACE inhibitors are considered once the patient has been stabilized, usually on day 3–5.

77. a. True
b. False
c. False
d. False
e. True

Comment: Diabetes mellitus is not a contraindication to thrombolysis; however, thrombolysis is contraindicated in the presence of proliferative diabetic retinopathy. Blood pressure can be reduced with intravenous glyceryl trinitrate. Thrombolysis can be repeated with recombinant tissue plasminogen activator, but not with streptokinase.

78. a. True
b. True
c. True
d. False
e. True

Comment: Ventricular ectopics rarely require treatment; however, β-blockers are the drugs of choice if treatment is needed.

79. a. False
b. False
c. True
d. False
e. True

Comment: Torsades de pointes is a variant of ventricular tachycardia with the potential to degenerate into VF cardiac arrest; it usually requires urgent management. Amiodarone and many other antidysrhythmic drugs can prolong the QT interval and, therefore, are not indicated in the treatment of torsades de pointes.

80. a. True
b. False
c. False
d. False
e. True

Comment: Capture and fusion beats are a feature of VT. Verapamil can be hazardous in VT and should never be used to differentiate between VT and SVT with BBB.

81. a. False
b. True
c. False
d. True
e. False

Comment: For pulseless VT a non-synchronized DC shock is administered. Atropine (3 mg) is given once as a bolus in asystole. BLS is essential in all settings in and out of hospital.

82. a. True
b. True
c. True
d. True
e. True

Comment: Remember 4 Hs and 4 Ts.

83. a. False
b. False
c. True
d. True
e. False

Comment: The AV node is supplied by the circumflex artery in 10% of patients. Following anterior myocardial infarction, AV node disorders are usually irreversible. Many patients with third-degree AV block are asymptomatic, but they still require permanent pacing.

84. a. True
b. True
c. False
d. False
e. False

Comment: Symptomatic bradycardia due to β-blockers usually responds to withdrawing the drug; temporary pacing may be needed until the drug effect is worn out. Left bundle branch block is not an indication for permanent pacing unless there is evidence of associated AV node disorder or heart failure. AV node disorders can be reversible up to 2 weeks after inferior myocardial infarction.

85. a. True
b. False
c. False
d. True
e. False

Comment: LBBB is associated with M-shaped complexes in V6. Atropine does not affect rhythm disturbances that originate below the AV node. LBBB is usually asymptomatic unless associated with AV node disease.

86.
a. True
b. False
c. True
d. False
e. True

Comment: In atrial fibrillation the random electrical atrial activity cannot be sensed and, therefore, dual-chamber pacing is not indicated. Pacemaker syndrome occurs with single-chamber pacemakers implanted in patients with atrial activity.

87.
a. True
b. True
c. False
d. False
e. True

Comment: Nitrates should be given intravenously as an infusion in acute left-ventricular failure. β-Blockers are introduced only after the patient is stabilized and free from both pulmonary and peripheral oedema.

88.
a. True
b. False
c. True
d. True
e. False

Comment: Amyloidisis and sarcoidosis cause infiltrative myocardial diseases and restrictive cardiomyopathy.

89.
a. True
b. True
c. True
d. True
e. False

Comment: Nitrates and other vasodilators increase outflow obstruction and are contraindicated in HCM.

90.
a. True
b. True
c. False
d. False
e. True

Comment: The heart is not enlarged unless there is associated pericardial effusion. Echocardiography is usually normal.

91.
a. True
b. True
c. False
d. True
e. False

Comment: Dressler's syndrome usually occurs 7–14 days after acute myocardial infarction. Treatment is usually with non-steroidal anti-inflammatory agents; corticosteroids are rarely needed.

92.
a. False
b. True
c. True
d. True
e. True

Comment: Pulsus paradoxus is a feature of cardiac tamponade.

93.
a. True
b. False
c. False
d. True
e. True

Comment: The pericardial rub usually disappears as pericardial effusion develops. Sinus tachycardia and not bradycardia is a feature of tamponade.

94.
a. False
b. False
c. True
d. True
e. True

Comment: Rheumatic fever can affect all heart valves. Valvular pathology is an autoimmune process (Aschoff nodule) triggered by pharyngeal infection with group A β-haemolytic streptococci.

95.
a. True
b. True
c. True
d. True
e. False

Comment: A negative blood culture suggests neither success nor failure of treatment; however, a positive culture is a sign of failure of treatment.

96.
a. True
b. False
c. True
d. True
e. True

Comment: *Staphylococcus aureus* infection can be rapid and destructive; therefore, every attempt must be made to treat the infection with appropriate antibiotics for the proper duration.

97.
a. True
b. True
c. True
d. True
e. False

Comment: Non-pharmacological management of hypertension is essential in all patients, and helps to reduce both systolic and diastolic blood pressure.

98.
a. True
b. True
c. False
d. True
e. False

Comment: Early diastolic murmur suggests aortic valve incompetence, which is not usually caused by hypertension. LBBB is usually secondary to ischaemic heart disease and is not a feature of hypertension.

99. a. False
    b. True
    c. False
    d. True
    e. False

Comment: Pulmonary artery pressure is usually low because pulmonary stenosis protects the pulmonary circulation. Patent ductus arteriosus is not a feature of tetralogy of Fallot. Total surgical correction includes closure of any right-to-left shunts.

100. a. True
     b. False
     c. True
     d. True
     e. False

Comment: Eisenmenger's syndrome is associated with polycythaemia and is irreversible.

SAQ answers

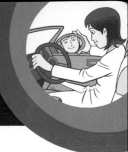

1. Management of acute pulmonary oedema includes:
   - Sit the patient up.
   - Administer oxygen (100%) via a facial mask.
   - Establish intravenous access and administer the following: diamorphine 2.5–5 mg; metoclopramide 10 mg; furosemide (frusemide) 80 mg.
   - Insert a urethral catheter.
   - Consider the need for intravenous nitrate infusion.
   - Continue to monitor the patient with regular measurements of blood pressure and blood oxygen saturation.

2. Investigations for patient with chest pain:
   - A full blood count – to exclude anaemia, which can precipitate angina. A patient who has pneumonia or a myocardial infarction may have a leucocytosis.
   - Urea and electrolytes – to show any renal impairment that may affect subsequent drug therapy or may worsen if the patient is hypotensive. Hypokalaemia is an important cause of arrhythmias in patients after myocardial infarction.
   - Liver function tests and amylase – may be abnormal if the chest pain is due to cholecystitis or pancreatitis.
   - Cardiac troponin – if elevated suggest acute myocardial infarction, if negative this investigation should be repeated 12 h after onset of symptoms. This is a sensitive marker of myocardial ischaemia – and a positive result may confirm the diagnosis and help in risk stratification of the patient
   - Electrocardiogram – this may show ST segment depression in angina or regional ST elevation in myocardial infarction. Global ST elevation that is saddle shaped suggests pericarditis. If large a pulmonary embolus may result in the classic S1, Q3, T3 appearance.
   - Chest radiograph – may show pulmonary oedema in a patient who has a myocardial infarction. Pulmonary embolus may produce a region of oligaemia on the chest film. Widening of the mediastinum suggests aortic dissection.

3. Clinical features of syncope:
   - The precipitating factors – may point to a cause (e.g. painful stimuli suggests a vasovagal cause).
   - Speed of onset is important – sudden onset suggests a cardiac or cerebrovascular cause whereas gradual onset suggests a metabolic cause.
   - Presence or absence of warning signs – cardiac syncope usually occurs without warning whereas epilepsy and hypoglycaemia are usually preceded by specific symptoms.

   - Witness account of the period of unconsciousness – specifically the presence of tonic–clonic movements, tongue biting or incontinence, all of which suggest epileptiform seizures.
   - Speed and nature of recovery – cardiac syncope is usually followed by a rapid recovery, but a patient will often be very drowsy after an epileptic seizure.

4. Complications of AFib:
   - Complications secondary to persistent tachycardia, which may lead to cardiac failure. Angina may also be exacerbated by the tachycardia.
   - Complications secondary to thromboembolism. The stasis of blood within the atria may lead to intracardiac clot formation and subsequent embolization may manifest as stroke, mesenteric infarction, or infarction of the fingers or toes.

5. Signs of endocarditis:
   - Hands – splinter haemorrhages, clubbing, Osler's nodes, Janeway lesions.
   - Skin – vasculitic rash.
   - Urine – microscopic haematuria.
   - Eyes – Roth's spots, conjunctival haemorrhages.
   - Neurological system – focal neurological defect.
   - Peripheral infarcts.
   - Joints – arthritis and swelling.

6. What does this ECG show?
   - Atrial flutter with slow ventricular response (4 to 1 block).
   - Treatment options include DC cardioversion with a synchronized shock – the patient should be fully anticoagulated with warfarin for at least 3 months to reduce the risk of thromboembolism. Cardioversion using drug therapy could be attempted using class III antiarrhythmic agents, such as sotalol or amiodarone, but these may slow the ventricular rate further, resulting in hypotension secondary to profound bradycardia.
   - As the ventricular rate is already slow, rate control using class II or IV agents is not indicated.
   - In all cases the underlying cause for the atrial flutter should be sought and treated.
   - Radiofrequency ablation is an option for refractory cases.

7. Investigations for suspected infective endocarditis:
   - Blood tests – six sets of blood cultures must be performed at least 1 h apart before antibiotics are started if the patient is well enough.

- A full blood count is performed to look for a leucocytosis and for anaemia of chronic disease.
- Urea and electrolytes will exclude renal failure, which may be a consequence of endocarditis and may influence the drug therapy. Liver function may be deranged in sepsis.
- Chest radiograph – this may show evidence of left-ventricular failure.
- Electrocardiogram – there may be a sinus tachycardia. Heart block is an extremely serious sign and suggests the presence of a septal abscess.

8. What does this ECG show:

- Complete heart block.
- Possible causes include inferior myocardial infarction, drug therapy (especially with antiarrhythmic agents), congenital complete heart block, septal abscess, aortic valve replacement.

9. Complications of cardiac catheterization:

- Complications involving the puncture site include haemorrhage, excessive bruising and pseudoaneurysm formation. The puncture site may become infected.
- The artery used for access may become thrombosed resulting in an ischaemic leg or arm.
- Trauma caused by the catheter may result in embolization of pieces of plaque to the cardiac, cerebral, or peripheral circulation causing myocardial infarction, cerebrovascular event, ischaemic toes or hands, or mesenteric infarcts.
- Myocardial or coronary artery tears may occur resulting in haemopericardium and possibly pericardial tamponade.
- Anaphylactic reactions to the dye used may occur and in some cases are fatal.

10. What does this figure show?

- The patient has developed ventricular tachycardia.
- See Fig. 5. It is very important that you know the algorithms for basic and advanced life support (see also Figs 13.1 and 13.4).

11. Signs of mitral stenosis:

- The patient may be dyspnoeic.
- The patient may have a malar flush.
- The patient may be in atrial fibrillation so the pulse is irregularly irregular.
- The apex beat is not displaced and is tapping in nature.
- There may be a loud first heart sound.
- There is an opening snap after the second heart sound followed by a low rumbling mid-diastolic murmur heard best at the apex with the patient lying on his or her left side and in full expiration.
- If pulmonary hypertension has developed there is a loud pulmonary component of the second heart sound (P2) and a left parasternal heave.
- If the pulmonary hypertension has led to right-ventricular impairment, the jugular venous pressure will be elevated and there will be peripheral oedema, ascites and hepatomegaly. There may be tricuspid regurgitation.

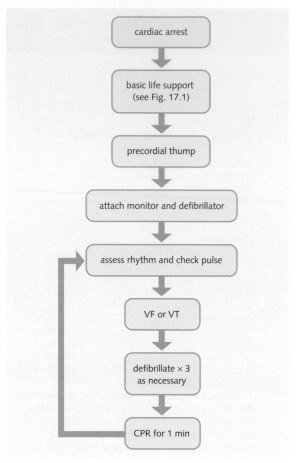

Fig. 5

12. What is shown in Fig. 4:

- Anteroseptal myocardial infarction.
- There are no Q waves; therefore the onset must have been less than 24 h previously.

13. Clinical signs of patent ductus arteriosus:

- A patent ductus arteriosus occurs if there is failure of the closure of the fetal connection between the pulmonary artery and the aorta after birth. Blood, therefore, passes from the high-pressure aorta into the lower-pressure pulmonary system, creating a left-to-right shunt.
- If the shunt is large the child may be breathless due to left-ventricular failure and there is failure to thrive, so the child may be small and underweight.
- On examination the pulse is collapsing in nature and of high volume.
- The cardiac apex is thrusting and may be displaced downward and laterally if there is left-ventricular failure. There is a palpable thrill at the second left intercostal space. On auscultation at the same place there is a loud continuous machinery murmur obscuring the second heart sound.

- If the shunt is large and pulmonary hypertension develops there may be reversal of the shunt and Eisenmenger's syndrome occurs – this causes differential cyanosis (cyanosed feet and pink hands) and usually develops after several years so is unlikely to be seen in a young child.

14. Investigations for ankle oedema:
    - Full blood count – anaemia can precipitate cardiac failure and is also seen in other disease (e.g. renal impairment, hypothyroidism).
    - Renal function (urea and electrolytes) – renal impairment may cause ankle oedema. Patients who have long-standing cardiac or hepatic impairment often have deranged renal function.
    - Liver function tests – deranged in hepatic failure.
    - Plasma albumin concentration – reduced in protein-losing states, such as nephrotic syndrome or protein-losing gastroenteropathy, but also reduced in any chronic disease state.
    - Thyroid function tests – hyperthyroidism may precipitate cardiac failure.
    - In addition to these baseline tests it may be appropriate to exclude Cushing's disease by performing cortisol measurements and a dexamethasone suppression test.

15. 60-year-old male:
    - The pain described is classically pericarditic and in a patient 6 weeks after a myocardial infarction suspect Dressler's syndrome as being the diagnosis. Dressler's syndrome is also associated with pleurisy (which would explain the bilateral pleural effusions) and arthritis.
    - The main differential diagnoses would be:
      ◦ pericarditis of another cause (e.g. viral causes such as coxsackie virus and enterovirus)
      ◦ pulmonary embolus – must be considered in any patient who is breathless after an illness
      ◦ pneumonia – especially if the organism is atypical (e.g. mycoplasma) – may also cause chest pain on breathing, pleural effusions, arthralgia and a low-grade fever

16. 40-year-old publican:
    - The symptoms suggest a diagnosis of congestive cardiac failure – suggested by dyspnoea, orthopnoea and oedema.
    - The most likely cause is chronic heavy alcohol consumption resulting in alcoholic cardiomyopathy.
    - Other possible causes are ischaemic heart disease and haemochromatosis.

17. Write short notes on streptokinase:
    - Streptokinase is a protein derived from β-haemolytic streptococci.
    - It has been shown to reduce the mortality rate in patients who have acute myocardial infarction when given within 24h of the onset of pain.
    - Streptokinase acts by binding to plasminogen to form a complex that activates to convert another molecule of plasminogen to plasmin. This results in fibrinolysis and breakdown of thrombus. Streptokinase acts on all plasminogen – it is not clot specific.
    - The drug is given as a 1-h intravenous infusion of 1.5 million units.
    - It has a half-life of 18min, but the complex with plasminogen has a half-life of 180min.
    - Side effects and complications of streptokinase include anaphylaxis, hypotension and haemorrhage.
    - Antibody production to the drug renders subsequent doses less effective; therefore, many centres will not use streptokinase more than once in the same patient.

18. Complications in the first 7 days following myocardial infarction:
    - Cardiac complications include:
      ◦ cardiac arrhythmias (including ventricular and supraventricular tachyarrhythmias and heart block)
      ◦ cardiac failure
      ◦ myocardial rupture including the septum or free wall
      ◦ papillary muscle rupture resulting in torrential mitral regurgitation.
    - Non-cardiac complications include:
      ◦ pulmonary embolus and deep venous thrombosis
      ◦ thromboembolic stroke secondary to mural thrombus formation
      ◦ haemorrhagic stroke secondary to thrombolysis adminstration
      ◦ pneumonia.

19. Indications for PPM:
    - See Fig. 14.8, p. 119.

20. A young woman attends:
    - See Fig. 19.3, p. 162.
    - The most important aspect to stress is that any dental work, even a session with the hygienist, requires antibiotic cover.
    - Other invasive procedures requiring cover include operations of any sort and cystoscopy.
    - The simplest and most effective piece of advice to give is to ensure that all medical and dental professionals who see the patient are advised of the medical condition from the start.

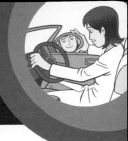
1.

1. (d) Prolonged QT interval (corrected for heart rate – QTc) on the ECG may suggest long QT syndrome, which is an inheritable condition that predisposes to sudden cardiac death, as it becomes more likely that the ensuing R wave will occur at the same time as the T wave of the previous complex. This can give rise to the so-called 'R on T' phenomenon, which may lead to torsades de pointes.

2. (e) Widespread concave or saddle-shaped ST elevation occurs in pericarditis. This may be confused with ST elevation from acute myocardial infarction; however, they may be distinguished by the history and examination findings and the fact that changes on the ECG due to pericarditis do not usually correspond to a coronary territory. If in doubt an echocardiogram is helpful.

3. (c) Other possible voltage criteria for LVH include tall R wave >25 mm in V5–V6, tall R wave >20 mm in lead II, and there may be T wave inversion in I, AVL, V5 and V6.

4. (j) Due to fluid accumulation around the heart, the voltage on the ECG is reduced, giving rise to smaller complexes. (This may also occur if the body mass index is raised.) Movement of the heart within the pericardial fluid can give rise to electrical alternans, whereby the complexes are of varying size in the same ECG lead recording.

5. (g) ST elevation in the inferior leads (II, III and AVF) suggests inferior MI. The ST depression in V2–V4 suggests posterior infarction, which occasionally occurs in isolation (so-called 'true posterior MI'). Of course ST depression in V2–V4 may reflect LAD territory ischaemia involving the anterior wall of the left ventricle.

2.

1. (e) Rhythm control strategy is the aim of maintaining sinus rhythm. Numerous drugs are capable of this, the chance of success depending on duration of AF, LV function, mitral valve disease and left atrial size. A standard β-blocker should be the initial treatment option. Caution should be taken with sotalol as it also has class III effects of prolonging the QT interval, so ECG monitoring is necessary. Digoxin is effective only for rate control of AF and flecainide is to be avoided in the presence of coronary artery disease or poor LV function.

2. (d) β-blockers are contraindicated in asthma, so both atenolol and sotalol are ruled out. Flecainide is effective, but must be avoided in heart failure or coronary artery disease. Amiodarone is an alternative but is best avoided in young patients due to long-term toxicity and side effects.

3. (g) These agents are also effective in SVT prophylaxis as they slow conduction through the AV node and by altering the refractory period of tissues can interfere with the re-entry circuit. However, digoxin and verapamil should be avoided if there is an accessory pathway; this is because blocking the AV node will then encourage conduction by the accessory pathway instead.

4. (j) Patients with VT and poor LV function should be considered for implantable cardioverter defibrillator with or without biventricular pacing (CRT). Both β-blockers and amiodarone may reduce the frequency of VT, but are inferior treatments to ICD therapy. As an adjunct to device therapy, if tolerated, β-blockers may be beneficial in heart failure and are, therefore, preferable to amiodarone.

5. (h) First-line rate control for AF should be with a β-blocker or rate-limiting calcium channel antagonist. Digoxin is less effective as it has poor control of exercise-related tachycardia.

3.

1. (i) Atenolol and amlodipine are both suitable options for the treatment of both angina and hypertension. However, atenolol has been superseded as a first-line treatment for hypertension alone.

2. (g) ACE inhibitors and ARBs are suitable options in diabetic patients with hypertension. However, this patient describes a well-recognized side effect of ACE inhibitors and should, therefore, be changed onto an ARB.

3. (d) Methyldopa is a centrally acting antihypertensive agent that is often used to treat hypertension in pregnancy. β-blockers are used in pregnancy. Pre-eclampsia should be excluded in this patient.

4. (h) The first choice antihypertensive agent in an AfroCaribbean patient should be either a calcium channel blocker or a diuretic.

5. (f) First-line treatment in this patient would either be a calcium channel antagonist or a diuretic. However, the diuretic is likely to exacerbate her urinary symptoms (urinary tract infection having been excluded) and, therefore, amlodipine is preferable; otherwise she is likely not to be compliant!

4.

1. (b) This man has a history that is compatible with angina. The first-line investigation is an exercise stress test, which will give information about his exercise capacity and symptoms, heart rate and blood pressure response to exercise, and whether any ischaemic ECG changes are seen in association with his symptoms. If this test is positive for inducible ischaemia then the next step is coronary angiography.
2. (g) The history suggests a problem regarding structural heart disease and this is best investigated in the first instance with an echocardiogram.
3. (f) This patient has a high probability of significant coronary artery disease and there is objective evidence of ischaemia. He should have coronary angiography to evaluate his coronary anatomy and establish whether revascularization is necessary, and if so by what means (i.e. angioplasty/stenting or CABG).
4. (i) This lady's symptoms are not typical of myocardial ischaemia, but this needs to be excluded given her risk factors. She is unlikely to be able to undergo exercise stress testing and, therefore, an alternative non-invasive assessment is appropriate. Either a stress echocardiogram or myocardial perfusion scan is reasonable.
5. (h) A 24-h ECG is likely to document the cause of her palpitations as her symptoms occur on a daily basis.

5.

1. (g) This man is known to have coronary artery disease and in view of his history we would expect that his left-ventricular function is reduced due to damage from previous myocardial infarctions. The scar tissue predisposes him to ventricular tachycardia, which may well cause him to lose consciousness. An ICD is indicated if this is proven.
2. (e) Dizziness on standing is suggestive of postural hypotension. This is often due to vasodilator antihypertensive drugs, but in this case may also be due to autonomic neuropathy as a result of her diabetes.
3. (c) The heart rate suggests complete heart block and his symptoms are compatible with this. An ECG will confirm the diagnosis.
4. (a) The clinical findings and family history suggest HCM. An echocardiogram and Holter monitor should be performed.
5. (f) Vasovagal syncope is most likely in a patient of this age and in this context. It should be confirmed from the history, examination and ECG that no other cause is being overlooked.

6.

1. (d) This patient has heart valve disease resulting from previous rheumatic fever. Endocarditis is likely to have resulted from a bacteraemia, such

as that resulting from dental work. Therefore, antibiotic prophylaxis is recommended prior to dental or other invasive procedures.
2. (a) Glomerulonephritis results from a type III autoimmune reaction, in which soluble immune complexes (aggregations of antigen and IgG or IgM antibodies) are deposited in tissues such as the kidney and triggers the classical pathway of complement activation.
3. (j) Libman-Sacks endocarditis is seen in patients with systemic lupus erythematosus and is not related to infection. Microbes that cause endocarditis and negative blood cultures include *Bartonella, Coxiella, Chlamydia, Legionella* and *Brucella* species as well as fungi and the HACEK group (*Haemophilus* species, *Actinobacillus actinomycetemcomitans, Cardiobacterium hominis, Eikenella corrodens* and *Kingella kingae*). Blood cultures may also be negative if antibiotics have been started before blood cultures are taken.
4. (b) It is notoriously difficult to eradicate infection from prosthetic heart valves. The fastidiousness of the organism also plays an important part. It is extremely important to work closely with the microbiology department.
5. (f) Roth's spots are retinal haemorrhages that may result from infective endocarditis.

7.

1. (f) This is the typical feature of RBBB.
2. (e) Complete heart block is exemplified by p waves which 'march' through the rhythm strip with no relationship to the QRS complexes. A ventricular escape rhythm is usually 30–40 beats per minute and gives rise to wide QRS complexes.
3. (g) J waves are pathognomonic of hypothermia.
4. (h) δ waves arise from the 'pre-excitation' of the ventricular myocardium. This results from antegrade conduction via the accessory pathway. The accessory pathway differs from the AV node in that it does not have a regulatory 'slowing down' function. Therefore, the PR interval is shortened.
5. (c) Accelerated idioventricular rhythm is a broad complex automatic ventricular rhythm, which commonly occurs in the first 48 h following a myocardial infarction. It rarely causes compromise and often reflects successful reperfusion of the myocardium. It is distinguished from VT as the heart rate is less than 120 bpm.

8.

1. (g) The clinical findings following trauma suggest tension pneumothorax. This is a clinical diagnosis and if untreated will result in cardiovascular collapse. It is treated without performing a chest X-ray by aspiration and insertion of a chest drain.
2. (c) The differential diagnosis includes pericardial effusion, pulmonary embolus, chest infection

and silent MI. The lack of chest pain or cough and the history of metastatic cancer point towards pericardial effusion and this needs to be investigated and treated urgently. The JVP may be elevated and there may be Kussmaul's sign (paradoxical increase in the JVP with inspiration). Pulsus paradoxus can be detected clinically by measuring the blood pressure with inspiration. It is important to exclude a pericardial effusion before giving heparin or warfarin to cover for PE, as this may make a pericardial effusion much worse!

3. (a) This man is compromised with hypotension secondary to complete heart block. The offending drug(s) should be discontinued and it is likely that he will need a permanent pacemaker (if complete heart block persists once the drug has washed out). In the meantime as he is symptomatic a temporary pacing wire should be inserted.

4. (i) The history suggests pericarditis caused by a viral infection. The symptoms and ECG changes are not suggestive of ischaemia. The most important complication of this is involvement of the myocardium which can lead to impairment of ventricular function, or pericardial effusion causing haemodynamic compromise. Rarely pericardial constriction may result in the long term.

5. (e) This lady has had a pulmonary embolus until proven otherwise! She should receive treatment dose low-molecular-weight heparin and be investigated either with a VQ scan (perfusion only) or CTPA – after discussion with the radiologist.

9.

1. (b) This gentleman should also be started on an ACE inhibitor, as long as there is no contraindication. This has been shown to reduce mortality in large randomized clinical trials (SAVE/HOPE /TRACE studies). The renal function should be monitored.

2. (b) The next step in this lady's management is the introduction of an ACE inhibitor. ACE inhibitors have been shown to reduce both morbidity and mortality in patients with heart failure (CONSENSUS/ /SOLVD studies). The mechanism of benefit is thought to be attenuation of the renin-angiotensin-aldosterone axis, which mediates the neurohormonal response to heart failure.

3. (f) Spironolactone should be introduced next. This is proven to be of benefit in patients with NYHA class 3 or 4 symptoms due to heart failure (RALES study). Monitoring of the renal function is necessary.

4. (h) Patients who do not benefit from conventional first line therapy may benefit from hydralazine and nitrate in combination. This was demonstrated in African Americans in the A-HeFT study.

5. (a) This patient should be started on a β-blocker with the aim of reducing his heart rate to 60 bpm. There is good evidence that this reduces mortality after MI (ISIS-1 study).

10.

1. (i) This patient is likely to have significant coronary artery disease, which may be amenable to angioplasty and stent treatment, or alternatively may require coronary artery bypass grafting.

2. (g) If the patient is compromised then even if the rhythm is SVT they should still be managed with DC cardioversion.

3. (f) This patient is not compromised despite ventricular tachycardia. Therefore, cardioversion can be attempted with electrolyte supplementation and amiodarone via a central venous catheter. This patient will obviously require further investigation in order to exclude myocardial ischaemia as a cause and evaluate LV function with a view to consideration of device therapy.

4. (e) This patient requires a permanent pacemaker as they are at risk of syncope or even ventricular standstill.

5. (j) Management is likely to include frusemide, oxygen, intravenous nitrates and opiates if tolerated, and non-invasive ventilation (NIV) such as continuous positive airway pressure (CPAP) if necessary. Anaesthetic input may be required and is best sought early!

11.

1. (d) Amlodipine can cause ankle swelling, and if this is troublesome, an alternative antihypertensive should be used instead. Alternatively, if another treatment is needed to control the blood pressure then the addition of a diuretic may resolve the ankle swelling.

2. (g) Acute deterioration in renal function may result if the patient has renal artery stenosis. This is because the efferent renal arteriole is preferentially dilated compared to the afferent arteriole, so the perfusion pressure across the kidney falls.

3. (i) A rash may result as a reaction to the contrast agent used for the angiogram, or as a reaction to clopidogrel. If the former is responsible, symptoms will resolve. If clopidogrel is the cause of the rash this may resolve with time. The clopidogrel should not be discontinued without discussion with a consultant cardiologist, as this may predispose to acute stent thrombosis, which is potentially fatal.

4. (b) ISMN often causes headaches and if not tolerated should be discontinued. In favour of an alternative antianginal.

5. (c) Erectile dysfunction is a well-recognized side effect of β-blockers and unless essential can be discontinued – a calcium channel antagonist, such as verapamil or diltiazem, is often prescribed instead.

12.

1. (k) Trisomy 21 is associated with several congenital heart lesions and one or more of these occur in approximately 40% of cases.

2. (j) Maternal rubella can cause a patent (also called persistent) ductus arteriosus and pulmonary stenosis as well as cataracts, deafness and microcephaly.

3. (l) The two most common cardiovascular malformations are bicuspid aortic valve (which can lead to aortic stenosis) and aortic coarctation – both obstructive lesions. Partial anomalous venous drainage and aortic dilatation are recognized, but less common.

4. (h) Because of the underlying connective tissue abnormalities, aortic root dilatation is a relatively common finding and predisposes to aortic dissection. Valve regurgitation may also occur, usually affecting the aortic or mitral valves.

5. (i) Kartagener's syndrome involves dextrocardia (or situs inversus – transposition of the viscera) as well as bronchiectasis and sinusitis.

13.

1. (b) A left parasternal heave indicates pulmonary hypertension. The right ventricle sits anteriorly and this is under strain against an increased pulmonary artery pressure.

2. (h) A double apical impulse suggest hypertrophic cardiomyopathy. The left ventricle is stiff and this results in raised left-ventricular end-diastolic pressure. Therefore, the left atrium has to contract forcefully and it is this impulse in addition to left-ventricular contraction that may be palpated.

3. (a) The regurgitant jet causes back pressure in the right atrium and this is transmitted to the venous system causing hepatic congestion and (if severe) pulsatile hepatomegaly.

4. (g) Obscuring of the second heart sound is indicative of severe aortic stenosis. Other clinical signs include an ejection systolic murmur, a thrill over the precordium, slow-rising or low-volume pulse and narrow pulse pressure.

5. (e) These signs are suggestive of mitral-valve prolapse. This is usually idiopathic, but may occur in association with connective-tissue disorders.

14.

1. (f) Hyperkalaemia is associated with tall T waves and short P wave amplitudes; the changes are dependent on the K^+ concentration. At higher concentrations, the PR interval becomes longer and QRS complexes become wider and eventually asystolic cardiac arrest occurs. Note that the ECG changes in hypokalaemia are the reverse with larger P wave and smaller T amplitudes leading to VT/VF as the terminal cardiac event.

2. (e) Widespread concave or saddle-shaped ST segment elevation occurs in pericarditis. Other ECH changes that may be seen include T wave inversion and atrial fibrillation.

3. (d) Long-standing hypertension leads to left-ventricular hypertrophy.

4. (g) The chest leads V1–V4 'look' at the anterior wall of the left ventricle. The presence of

Q waves supports the presence of old trans-mural myocardial infarction.

5. (a) The leads II. III and AVF 'look' at the inferior wall of the heart, and ST elevation on the ECG is seen in the acute phase of myocardial infarction.

15.

1. (c) Diabetic patients with ongoing ischaemia and three-vessel coronary artery disease will benefit prognostically and symptomatically from revascularization.

2. (d) These symptoms should be investigated, but in the absence of pre-syncope or syncope, and with a structurally normal heart it is unusual for any treatment to be required.

3. (b)

4. (g) Further symptomatic and prognostic benefit could be obtained with biventricular pacing.

5. (h) Familial hypercholesterolaemia needs to be excluded in this lady, who would benefit from specialist referral and family counselling. There is a high risk for the development of atheromatous vascular disease and, therefore, primary prevention is indicated.

16.

1. (g) Other side effects include hyperkalaemia, impotence and menstrual irregularities.

2. (c) Other side effects include flushing and postural hypotension.

3. (d) Myalgia is an important side effect of all statins and should always be investigated with serial assessments of creatinine kinase levels. A fourfold increase in the CK levels suggests that the drug should be discontinued. Liver biochemistry and function tests should also be monitored.

4. (a) This is in common with other β-blockers. Other side effects include broncho-spasm, bradycardia and erectile dysfunction.

5. (h) Bleeding with or without thrombocytopenia is a major side effect associated with the use of this glycoprotein IIa/IIIb inhibitor.

17.

1. (d) Rheumatic fever may result in rheumatic heart disease – most commonly affecting the mitral valve and causing mitral stenosis. The clinical signs are consistent with mitral stenosis. Atrial fibrillation is commonly seen in mitral stenosis – and is often a result of left atrial dilatation.

2. (g) Pulmonary hypertension as a result of chronic lung disease is known as *cor pulmonale.*

3. (c)

4. (h) Systemic sclerosis (scleroderma) and other autoimmune rheumatic disorders and vasculitidies are an important cause of pulmonary hypertension.

5. (i) This is a clinical scenario of pulmonary embolism, recent immobilization and typical symptoms.

18.

1. (c) These signs are consistent with aortic stenosis. Displacement of the apex beat suggests that there may be left-ventricular dilatation.
2. (b) The signs are of aortic regurgitation.
3. (j) The murmur described is that of mitral valve prolapse – in this instance surgical treatment may be warranted.
4. (g) Other causes of dilated cardiomyopathy include idiopathic, excess alcohol and post-partum.
5. (f) Systemic hypertension is an important cause of heart failure.

19.

1. (c) A young patient with severe LV dysfunction and stage IV heart failure, despite maximal medical therapy. This patient should be referred for consideration of heart transplantation.
2. (i) In patients with left main stem stenosis, current evidence supports CABG surgery as the treatment of choice.
3. (l) Cardiac arrhythmia is a common complication of myocardial infarction. In the absence of cardio-vascular instability (hypotension, collapse), it is safe to observe such arrhythmias for several days, in the assumption that they will resolve without treatment.
4. (j) This is an absolute indication for permanent pacemaker implantation.
5. (h) A coronary angiogram should be performed to determine the coronary artery anatomy, and help guide revascularization.

20.

1. (b) Over 90% of hypertension is 'essential', i.e. there is not treatable cause found.
2. (d) These symptoms are all consistent with a diagnosis of phaeochromcytoma. Hyperthyroidism is not normally associated with hypertension.
3. (g) The presence of a bruit in this area may suggest the presence of renal artery stenosis.
4. (i) Rib notching is a 'pathongomonic' sign of aortic co-arctation.
5. (a) Cushing's disease is caused by a primary pituitary adenoma, which may cause bitemporal hemianopia.

Index